FOUNDATION

FOREWORD BY LANCE ARMSTRONG

FOUNDATION

REDEFINE YOUR CORE, CONQUER BACK PAIN, AND MOVE WITH CONFIDENCE

DR. ERIC GOODMAN AND PETER PARK
WITH DIANE REVERAND

Rodale books may be purchased for business or promotional use or for special sales. For information, please write to: Special Markets Department, Rodale, Inc., 733 Third Avenue, New York, NY 10017

Printed in the United States of America
Rodale Inc. makes every effort to use acid-free ♾, recycled paper ♲.

Illustrations by Scott Holladay
Photographs by Elizabeth Kreutz
Page 9: Photo by Paul Mathieu

Book design by Christopher Rhoads

Library of Congress Cataloging-in-Publication Data
Goodman, Eric (Eric David), 1980–
    Foundation : redefine your core, conquer back pain, and move with confidence / Eric Goodman, Peter Park.
        p.   cm.
    ISBN 978–1–60961–100–2 paperback
    1. Backache—Popular works.   2. Backache—Exercise therapy—Popular works.   I. Park, Peter (Peter James), 1965–   II. Title.
    RD771.B217G66 2011
    617.5'64062—dc22   2011009112

Distributed to the trade by Macmillan

2   4   6   8   10   9   7   5   3   paperback

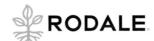

We inspire and enable people to improve their lives and the world around them.
www.rodalebooks.com

To our clients in Santa Barbara

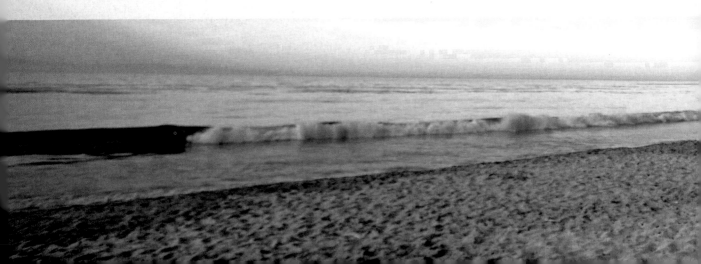

CONTENTS

FOREWORD BY
LANCE ARMSTRONG
FITNESS OFF THE BIKE

When I first came to Peter for help, I had a *lo-o-ong* way to go. I was 2 years into retirement and planned to spend the summer with my family in Santa Barbara. I was overweight from eating chips and burritos, food that was never part of my diet when I was racing. A mutual friend from Texas had introduced us a few years earlier, right after I had finished cancer treatment. I actually had known Peter for years. We would run into each other from time to time when my cycling teams visited the Santa Barbara area for training camps. Since he really knows endurance sports, I trusted him to know what I needed.

We started training together. Peter is one of the fittest people, if not *the* fittest person, I have ever been around. We worked together every day, focusing on the Chicago Marathon. I have to admit that there was a competitive element to the workouts. I did not like it when he could beat me in the gym or running on the trails in Santa Barbara. Lights started going off in my head as I did his unconventional exercises and felt the edge return. At first I thought I would never be able to get to a certain point, but I made constant progress with the workouts. I was amazed at how quickly I got to where I wanted to be. I started looking at the Tour de France.

His workouts were not traditional. I wasn't building strength by using weight machines and doing leg curls and squats. Instead, I was using gravity and body weight to strengthen my real core, the posterior chain of muscles—particularly the glutes and hamstrings—and to create flexibility and strength in my hips and lower back, teaching all of my muscles to work together.

When Peter joined forces with Eric, those exercises became even more targeted and far more powerful. By introducing Foundation training to my strength program, I was able to get back on the bike quickly with the same intensity I am known for. Training for the Tour de France always involves pain. Foundation training let me train hard while feeling great. My work with Peter and Foundation training is what started my comeback and is what will keep me fit off the bike.

INTRODUCTION

A SIMPLE PLAN

We have developed a new way for you to deal with your back pain that goes beyond treating your symptoms. If you have back pain, you want it to stop. You can (and probably have) achieved relief with medication and traditional rehabilitation. But often that approach provides a temporary fix. If you stop taking painkillers, your back will start bothering you again. The beneficial effects of physical therapy and massage last only so long. The reason you relapse is that these remedies don't get to the root of your back pain. Getting to the source of your pain is going to offer you more than a stopgap solution. It will enable you to move again with confidence and power.

It's no secret that our posture, sedentary lifestyle, and bad movement patterns put too much stress on the spine, particularly the lower spine, and the small back muscles. But when we created a program that redefined the core, shifting the emphasis from the abs to the much larger muscles in the back of the body, the result was the first practical solution to this long-standing dilemma. Foundation training is based on the simple but unique idea that strengthening the posterior chain allows the strong muscles in your back to do their job of supporting the weight of the upper body and propelling movement.

We joined forces to develop a series of exercises designed to change destructive movement patterns and build a powerful posterior chain, which begins with a strong lower back. The results we have seen in hundreds of clients have been

When we created a program that redefined the core, shifting the emphasis from the abs to the much larger muscles in the back of the body, the result was the first practical solution to this long-standing dilemma.

amazing. Our clients have been transformed by Foundation training, as you will see in the stories they tell throughout the book.

We feel so lucky to be able to make Foundation training available to all of you who are plagued and limited by back pain. We have seen what investing 20 to 40 minutes three times a week can do. The improvements our clients have experienced are so profound that they make Foundation training a way of life, and it has taken them to new levels of fitness. We know the simple exercises presented in this book will do the same for you.

Our goal is to give you three basic workouts of increasing intensity in the cleanest possible way. When we began to think about writing a book, we surveyed what was available. There was so much padding in many of the fitness books we read—

entirely too much extraneous information. Your goal is to end your back pain. We want to take you there directly. We would like to see you spending your time doing the workouts and applying your new energy to living well in all aspects of your life.

With Foundation training, you are building a solid muscular base. From there you can go anywhere with flexibility, power, and endurance. Once you learn to move properly, there are few limits to what you can achieve physically. Living without pain will boost your energy level and attitude. So get moving—the right way—and see how much better you will feel.

ERIC GOODMAN AND PETER PARK

THE BACKSTORY

1

WHEN WE FIRST TEAMED UP, WE KNEW WE WERE ONTO SOMETHING THAT WAS GOING TO HELP A LOT OF PEOPLE CONTEND WITH ONE OF THE MOST PERSISTENT AND DIFFICULT-TO-ANSWER QUESTIONS IN FITNESS AND HEALTH: **"HOW DO I GET OUT OF PAIN?"**

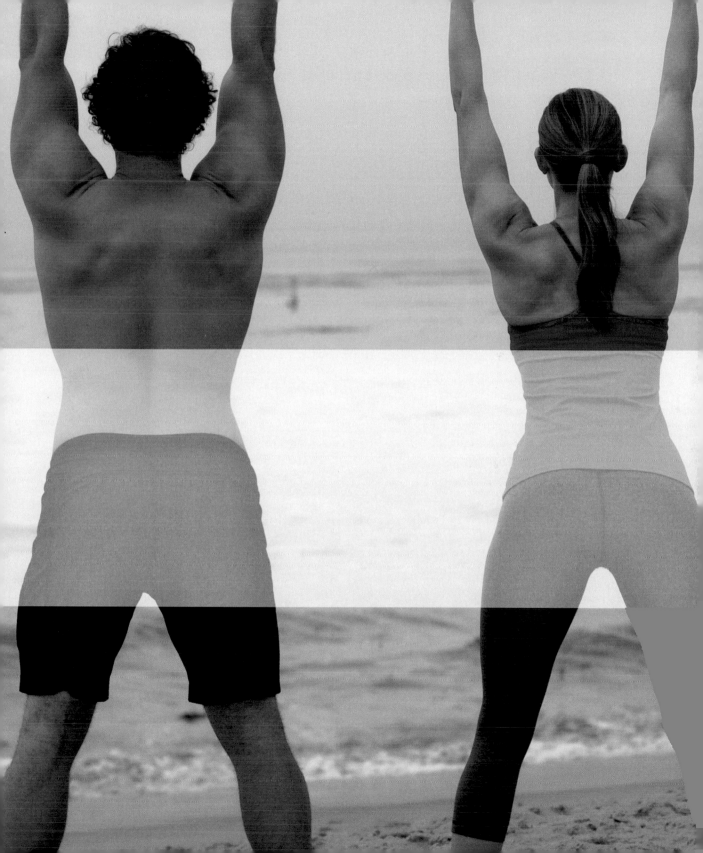

Our answer—one of the first new ideas to come about in the world of exercise in years—is Foundation training. Since we were offering something completely different, we did not know what to expect, but our simple workout has proven to be more effective than we could have imagined. The extent and speed of the improvements we see in our clients consistently surprise us. We could not have predicted what Foundation training is doing for people of any age at all levels of fitness. Based on the results we've seen, our motto has become *from pain to performance*.

Our confidence is confirmed daily by the dramatic changes in the lives of all the clients we are training. People who had tried everything to relieve their back pain began to feel a difference in as little as 2 weeks. Many of our clients had relied on prescription painkillers or over-the-counter remedies several times a day for years. They were happy to throw away those pill bottles and manage their pain with Foundation training. Others wanted to avoid surgery, and some were frustrated that going under the knife ultimately did not solve their back problems. They were so relieved to find that these exercises did more for them than extreme measures. Our success stories range from professional athletes, the likes of NBA legend Derek Fisher and world champion surfer Kelly Slater, to everyday people who

> Based on the results we've seen, our motto has become *from pain to performance.*

come to our weekly classes. We have seen remarkable changes in people from every walk of life. For example:

- After two back surgeries in 2 years, a client in his fifties was still stuck in debilitating back pain. He had almost forgotten what life was like without pain. In just 2 months of Foundation training, his pain was almost gone, and he was able to resume vigorous activities he had long ago given up.

- A mother of two showed no improvement with months of physical therapy after surgery to repair a herniated disc. She made great progress in a few short weeks with Foundation training. She's such a convert that she invites family and friends to join her one-on-one training sessions.

- Derek Fisher, point guard for the 2010 NBA Champs, the Los Angeles Lakers, had an impressive collection of injuries after 13 years of professional basketball. With Foundation training, he is in the best shape of his life, and he says his body feels better than it did in his early career.

- Pro surfer Kelly Slater used Foundation training to become pain free and powerful while competing for his 10th world championship surfing title.

- A larger-than-life financial genius had been taking powerful prescription painkillers twice a day for 2½ years after having many surgeries for his knees, back, and neck. After 8 months of Foundation training, he hikes 2 hours a day, paddleboards with his kids, and is completely off painkillers.

Our program produced unprecedented and lasting results. People were stronger, healthier, and feeling better than they ever thought they would again. Foundation training gave them a new quality of life, hope, and the tools to manage their pain and maximize their energy.

Our client list has grown exponentially. We never dreamed we would be working with so many influential people, movers and shakers in Hollywood, sports, and the business world. All this buzz, and we don't advertise or actively look for publicity. It has all been through word of mouth. When people break through the barriers that pain has created in their lives—often after years of trying—they want the world to know. Our clients can't seem to stop talking about what Foundation training has done for them.

Best of all, we get to write this book and to introduce Foundation training to everyone suffering from back pain who may not be lucky enough to live in Southern California, and that's a staggering number of people. More than 80 percent of the population of the United States and Europe will experience back pain in

FOUNDATIONFIRST

Derek Fisher, LA Laker and NBA champion

I search for the best of the best when it comes to my fitness and conditioning. I have always been in great shape and take pride in maintaining a certain level of fitness, but in the time I have been working with Peter Park and Eric Goodman, I have reached a new level of endurance, stamina, and strength. The program pushes me without exhausting me, conditions me, and has completely changed the way my body moves and feels.

their lifetimes. It's the most common reason people go to see a doctor, after upper-respiratory infections. Americans spend more than $50 billion a year on back pain. It does not have to be this way.

Foundation training is designed to strengthen your lower back and posterior chain; alleviate your back pain by correcting mechanical imbalances and weaknesses; and create maximum

> Foundation training redefines the core, shifting the focus from the abs and the front of the body to the back and the posterior chain.

power, flexibility, and endurance by concentrating on your real core. Foundation training redefines the core, shifting the focus from the abs and the front of the body to the back and the posterior chain. Before we explain in detail what Foundation training does for your body, we want to tell you how we arrived at this change of emphasis.

FOUNDATION ROOTS

Foundation training initially grew from Eric's experience, his education as a chiropractor, his own back problems, and his work as a trainer. He was an athlete, a personal trainer by age 18, but his movement patterns were all wrong and were actually creating injuries. He started to get back spasms at 19. It was painful for him to get up if he sat for a couple of hours, and he had to strain to stand up straight. The pain became more frequent each year he was in college. What started as discomfort was now creating a real problem. When he was a senior in college, he sat down at his computer to study after a long bike ride, and was gripped with pain that he'd never felt before; it was more severe than anything he'd ever experienced. When he tried to stand, his right leg went weak and just wouldn't work. A sharp pain shot into his spine and down his right leg. He lay down on his back on the floor with no idea of what was wrong. The pain radiated from very low in his back down the back of his right leg. He thought all the sports and exercises he had been doing were benefiting his body, but there he was flat out, unable to move without pain.

X-rays revealed that he had substantial dehydration of the discs and degeneration of the fourth and fifth lumbar vertebrae and the sacrum at the base of the spine. The discs were heavily compressed and severely degenerated. His last two vertebrae were sitting on top of each other. The x-rays showed the wear and tear of a much older spine. He hadn't even made it far into his twenties. His movement was inhibited because the muscles connected to his lower spine could not relax.

As Eric started chiropractic school, the pain persisted and worsened despite the fact that he could not have had better access to treatment. He was trying everything. He was getting adjusted frequently and had regular massages. Though treatments were effective for the short term, the pain always returned. For the next 3 years, there were very few days that he did not have some sort of back pain. He began to understand the ways in which pain can limit your life.

Eric observed that the baseline and plateau set by existing rehabilitation protocols were a bit too low. The fact is that 90 percent of people with back pain symptoms will feel better within 2 months, no matter what treatment is used, but the pain will return. Dealing with his own back problems, Eric found that traditional exercises and treatments seemed to have a ceiling on how much he improved; the results were less than stellar, and they were usually short-lived. It became obvious that the basic protocols and even doctoral-level training were not working for him; he had to believe that they were not working for other people, either. Eric became aware that much of the rehabilitation was based on movement patterns that were incorrect for our bodies. He realized that to stop pain for the long term, a fundamental change in movement had to occur. All the treatments and corrections he had been trying offered only a minimal shift in the mechanics of movement, and without that essential change, he would just keep reinjuring his back. He understood that the reason there is so much back, hip, and knee pain—that the statistics are so off the charts—is because we are loading our bodies incorrectly.

The reason there is so much back, hip, and knee pain is because we are loading our bodies incorrectly.

Eric had always been interested in Eastern medicine and philosophy, so he took up yoga to stay flexible and manage his pain. He studied Pilates, which focuses on the deep abdominal muscles and lower back, and modified his resistance training. He began to tweak yoga exercises in an attempt to strain and stress his body in slightly different ways. The exercises used torque and leverage to maximize the amount of tension on his weakest muscles. His goal was to build the deep supporting muscles of his spine. He wanted to concentrate all of the pull on the back side of his body; specifically, on the posterior chain—his neck, back, butt, hamstrings, and heels. With this shift in focus in mind, he developed the exercises of Foundation training, which are based on the essential principle that movement comes from the hip joints, using a braced spine and the posterior chain.

As Eric experimented with this new movement, his back started getting stronger, and the pain and uncertainty he had lived with for 4 years evaporated in a very short time. He began teaching his ideas to friends and a few patients. Around the same time he was asked to help Dr. Terry Schroeder with the USA Olympic water polo team as chiropractor and strength coach. Observing injuries the athletes were developing as a result of their demanding sport, Eric started to introduce modifications he was using himself into the team's training. He changed how people did standard exercises like squats and crunches, concentrating on the back of the body instead of the front. He worked with an entire team of Olympic athletes for nearly a year before the 2008 Games in Beijing.

FOUNDATIONFIRST

Tony Azevedo, USA water polo team captain, three-time Olympian, and "best athlete in the world 2004"

Ten months of Foundation training was one of the primary driving forces behind our team's winning the silver medal in Beijing in the 2008 Olympics. We were constantly called the strongest team in the water, even though we began the competition ranked number nine in the world.

The vast majority of those athletes responded extremely well to the changes in their workouts. The team remained injury free while performing at a high level through the months of tough training. Their bodies did not break down. The team exceeded everyone's expectations and went on to take the silver medal. It was one of the success stories of the Olympics. Eric has been fine-tuning the exercises ever since.

Eric moved to Santa Barbara in January 2009 and reached out to the fitness community there to establish himself. Among the people he contacted was a big name in fitness, Peter Park, an elite athlete and one of the most influential trainers in the world. He'd been Lance Armstrong's strength coach for more than 10 years.

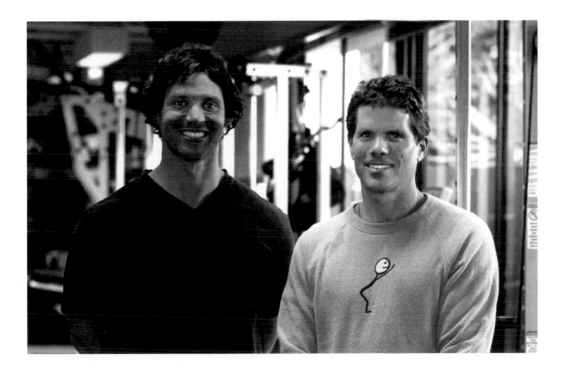

In his e-mail to Peter, Eric described the success he was having with Foundation training. Peter liked the sound of it. Even with his considerable experience, Peter had never heard of anything like Foundation. The rest is history.

We bounced our training philosophies off each other, and it was evident our ideas complemented each other very well. Eric visited Peter at one of his gyms to demonstrate his new approach. Peter was trying to remedy his own chronic back pain. Just as Eric had done, he was looking for answers and not finding them. We decided to train together for a while.

Peter didn't have any real injuries, but he was training at least 5 hours a day, which put a tremendous load on his joints. Over time, his movement patterns and the repeated stresses to his joints led to muscular imbalances. The pain he was experiencing was his body's way of warning, "Something's not right here. You need to change something."

We started with the basics. Peter was amazed by the results he experienced within a week or two. His body felt different—much more powerful. He noticed while running and biking that his back pain was diminished, and soon it disappeared. One of the best-trained athletes in the world had experienced a fundamental change in his movement patterns. He came to understand that the movements he had been working on for years and years just did not work. With the corrections provided by Foundation training, he found that his back and knees were hurting significantly less and the range of motion in his shoulders increased considerably. He became a different athlete after a few months of training.

Convinced that by combining forces we could really help people, we decided to partner up. Together, we have refined Foundation training with the goal of helping everyone at all levels of fitness to break through pain and exercise more effectively. Eric's focus is on fundamental movement patterns and building the initial strength needed to go forward. Peter works with clients to reinforce that strength and those movement patterns, bringing our clients to a pinnacle of fitness. Foundation training not only reduces pain but also opens a road map to fitness, giving people the tools to go wherever they want to go with assurance.

There is a reason we call it Foundation training. Learning these exercises will give you a strong structural foundation on which you can build, a baseline for any sport or exercise program. If you can create perfect movement for your body, everything else becomes so easy to do. With Foundation training at the center, you can branch out to whatever physical activity interests you—yoga, Pilates, P90X, weight lifting, tennis, golf, etc.

> With Foundation training at the center, you can branch out to whatever physical activity interests you—yoga, Pilates, P90X, weight lifting, tennis, golf, etc.

Our partnership has been 100 percent driven by results. Give us 2 weeks and you will notice a substantial difference in how you move. We are confident in saying this because we have seen these exercises work for so many people. We have helped young athletes, ages 13 to 15, whose parents had tried everything else to help their children resolve their back pain. Foundation training has allowed those young athletes to pursue their passion. We work with postsurgical clients in their forties, fifties, and sixties to bring them back to full mobility and an active life, and we have been able to steer many clients away from surgery and toward taking control of their pain, a fringe benefit of strengthening their backs. Peter even has two clients in their late eighties who continue to run and play tennis, doing what they've done their entire lives.

With this book, we want to reach beyond our immediate community to make Foundation available to people who need it—including many of you who are on your last nerve of chronic pain. Back pain is a barrier for millions of people, interfering with their health, happiness, and enjoyment of life. People come to us fed up with living in constant pain. After they incorporate the simple movements of Foundation training into their lives, it's not just their backs that feel better. They open up to a different idea of what their lives can be. They gain insight into how stressful the pain has been, affecting their moods and energy levels. Accustomed to being limited by pain, they are now energized by the realization that they can get out and do things without anxiety about further injuring themselves and bringing on more pain. They can once again enjoy their partners and kids as well as their own bodies. We have witnessed this transformation repeatedly. We want to give you our solution for back pain and help you accomplish powerful changes in your body and your life.

Foundation is a complete user's guide for the back and for your whole body. We want you to understand the central role your back plays in every move you make. Doing Foundation exercises just three times a week can significantly reduce the pain that has been dragging you down and inspire you to take control of your own wellness. We have designed a program of three workouts to be done progressively over 6 weeks. The workouts correspond to different levels of back pain and rehabilitation as well as difficulty: a basic workout for acute back pain, a moderate workout for chronic pain, and a more intense workout

Foundation is a complete user's guide for the back and for your whole body.

for prevention and strengthening during pain-free periods. As you cycle through the three levels, devoting 2 weeks to each level, you will not only reduce your pain but also feel stronger in everything you do. There is a bonus chapter of exercises for added flexibility, targeting tightness and pain in the hips, pelvis, and upper legs, a direct result of all the time people spend sitting.

The success of Foundation training is all in the results we see every day. Throughout the book, you'll read about what Foundation training has done for our clients. Their words are the best proof that this new approach to exercise works. Foundation training has reduced the pain and improved the fitness of every client we've worked with to date. We hope to count you as one of the growing number of people who have learned to manage their pain and raise their level of fitness with Foundation training.

Commit to doing these simple, equipment-free workouts three times a week and see how you feel. The only way you will know how effective these workouts are is to try them. You can do them anywhere, anytime. Don't wait. Start today.

REDEFINING THE CORE

2

THE NOTION THAT YOUR ABDOMEN IS THE CORE OF YOUR BODY IS DATED

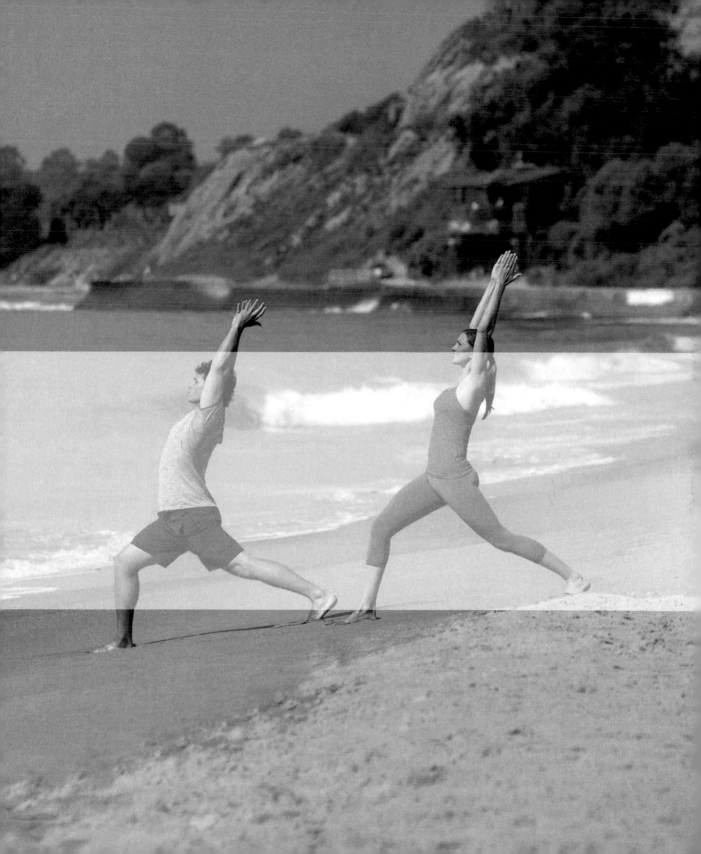

Most people have degeneration in their spines, but only some people are symptomatic, meaning they experience spasms and back pain. People are not aware of herniated discs and degeneration until the nerves in that area get inflamed. You know what we're talking about—it has happened to you or someone you know. Your back suddenly "goes out," and you are in excruciating pain with an acute condition that sends you to a doctor.

When you first learned that you had a herniated disc, you may have assumed that you did something that injured that part of your spine, but the degenerative process probably had been going on for years. The problem had been building because of repetitive,

> If you do not change your movement patterns, the injuries will progress and low-grade inflammation will persist.

mechanical stress on your spine. When most people move, every movement they make—forward bending, side bending, and each step—uses the wrong muscles and contributes to degeneration of the joints and spine. Acute pain will disappear for a time after traditional therapies, but if you do not change your movement patterns, the injuries will progress and low-grade inflammation will persist, resulting in chronic, nagging pain that restricts your activity and creates barriers in your life.

With Foundation training, we do not treat injuries. We teach your body, training it to move effectively, powerfully, and in balance so that injuries due to mechanical imbalances and weaknesses fall by the wayside. Conventional medicine, rehabilitation, and training address only the manifestations of the problem. Taking

FOUNDATIONFIRST

BACK TO HIS OLD SELF

When my husband, Ben, began Foundation training just a few years ago, his back pain was excruciating and his spirits were very low. All this was taking its toll on him and everyone around him. His pain was destructive to our family life.

Ben had suffered with debilitating back pain for more than 2 years. The simplest movement was impossible. The constant pain was diminishing him and causing him to wither under the agony. The suffering was written on his face. As each day passed, he was able to do less and less, which sunk his spirits to new lows. He was no longer able to enjoy our active family lifestyle. Many times he was in too much pain to participate in the activities we had planned. Darkness had come over our family. It was miserable.

Then we moved to Santa Barbara and discovered Foundation training. Within a very short time, I saw my husband smile again. The pained look on his face began to fade; he stopped taking megadoses of pain pills. He eventually discontinued even over-the-counter medicine. Soon we were taking walks on the beach, and, to my amazement, he progressed quickly to hiking trails with steep terrain. Our two sons, ages 9 and 14, had their father back. The dark cloud lifted, and the light brightened family life again. Foundation training gave us a modern-day miracle. Ben is doing great; he is pain free. Health is wealth, and we are joyful to have Ben back.

CHERYL TROSKY

painkillers is like putting a Band-Aid over the problem: Rather than getting to what is *causing* the pain, you are just trying to stop it. You can get a cortisone shot in your tennis elbow, and you might have relief for a few months. Sooner or later that pain will return, however, because you have not addressed what creates the pain. Our goal is to get to the root of the problem.

We do not treat injuries. We teach your body, training it to move effectively, powerfully, and in balance so that injuries due to mechanical imbalances and weaknesses fall by the wayside.

We have found that if you change the way you move, your pain will evaporate. We created Foundation training to correct damaging movement patterns and strengthen the muscles that keep your back stable.

Here's where redefining the core comes in.

The notion that your abdomen is the core of your body is dated. No matter what the problem, conventional wisdom says to strengthen your core: "You have to do situps; you have to do knee raises. And don't forget the crunches." The abs you see in the mirror—that six-pack everyone wants—may look good, but they have little to do with stability and movement. Traditional exercises used for rehabilitation hardly affect the spine. The thinking goes that you have to strengthen your abs to take some pressure off your spine. The truth is that focusing on your abs can actually weaken the back muscles that support and move your spine.

Muscle groups work in a balanced way. When one group fires, the other relaxes. If you bend forward, your back muscles lengthen and your abs contract. If you lean back from your waist or move your torso from side to side, your hip and abdominal muscles have to lengthen as your back muscles contract. All the muscles of the lower spine are constantly firing to maintain proper alignment of the vertebrae. The contraction of the ab muscles puts them under additional stress. When those muscles become fatigued or are subject to excess pressure, the result is back pain.

> For every exercise you do for the front of your body, you should do at least four for the back.

Foundation training makes conventional "core training" a thing of the past. Your abs are secondary to the back of your body. Foundation training shifts the emphasis to the back and the posterior chain, the deep supporting muscles that affect

THE SPIDERWEB THEORY

When a force is exerted on your core, it is felt throughout the entire body, just as every strand of a spiderweb responds to a touch on a single strand. Though it will not be as powerful or concentrated as where the initial force was made, the movement does affect the rest of the body. By strengthening the real core—which is, for us, the posterior chain—you will create a tangible impact in the movement of all the surrounding tissue, including your extremities.

every movement you make. The butt, hip, hamstring, back, and spine muscles are meant to generate more force than any other part of your body. We believe that for every exercise you do for the front of your body, you should do at least four for the back, because those muscles will provide you with powerful, pain-free movement.

Our hips are designed to be our central fulcrum, yet the way we live today restricts our natural movement by using the lower spine as our main mover. In the past, much of a person's time was spent in an upright position. Before industrialization, work was much more physical. Whether tending crops, hanging laundry, or kneading dough, we were putting variable pressures on the spine, which moved in all planes of motion. Today we drive everywhere; we sit at desks or conference tables at work; we spend the evenings in chairs watching TV, reading, or staring at computer screens. Our spines do not experience changes of position and stress. The stress on the spine is constant when we subject it to long periods of flexion or forward bending. These postures use the fragile lower back as the fulcrum and put a lot of pressure on that problem spot.

Our sedentary lifestyle is one reason back tightness and pain are so prevalent today. Not only does sitting for extended periods increase the pressure on your lower back, but a sedentary lifestyle can affect your circulation, depleting the back muscles of oxygen. After sitting at a computer for hours without moving, your muscles may suffer from oxygen deprivation. They will seize up, contracting dramatically. The result is a painful back spasm.

All that time hunched in our cars and at our desks means that we spend much

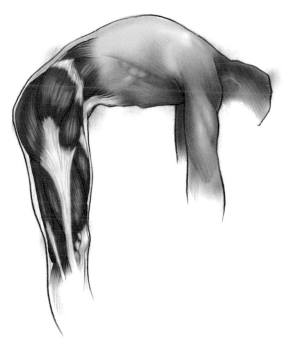

Wrong Movement Pattern—Flexed Spine

of our lives internally rotated—otherwise known as the computer syndrome—
which is only exacerbated by all those crunches. How often do you find yourself
standing with your neck forward, your shoulders slightly hunched, and your weight
shifted forward over your toes? That rotation is reinforced when we sit as much as
we do and work out with faulty movement patterns.

When the muscles in the front of your body contract, they pull your lower spine
forward. In order to do their job keeping the spine aligned, your spinal muscles
have to pull back. Internal rotation produces tension in the muscles at the back of
your body. Your hamstrings, upper and lower back, and neck all stay tight, and that

means overtaxed muscles and back pain. Working that hard can fatigue those muscles and create a back spasm. Instead of tightening the abdominal muscles, you need to relax them to reduce the pressure on your back. Bad posture and spending too much time immobile, either standing or sitting, mean that the forces of gravity are not evenly distributed on the muscles, ligaments, and bones of your spine, causing problems to develop.

When your spine is flexed or bent forward for long periods of time, you are stressing all the spinal structures, including the joints, ligaments, and muscles. Eventually, your body adapts to these stresses, resulting in the loss of mobility in

EFFORTLESS GOOD POSTURE

Nothing makes you look more confident, fit, and energetic than good posture. When your back is straight and you hold your head high, you look as if you are ready for anything. When you slouch, with your chest concave and your shoulders up to your ears, you look stressed and negative. You don't want to send that message.

The good news is that the most visible benefit of Foundation training is terrific posture—and you won't even have to think about it. When your spine is properly braced, your shoulders are automatically back, your chest is high as your spine curves naturally, and your movement originates in your hips.

Once you integrate Foundation exercises into your life, you won't have to think about posture, but here's a tip to start: If you want to improve your posture, pull your shoulder blades down, rather than back, to accentuate the natural curve of your spine.

your joints, degeneration in your joints, and changes in your discs.

Most exercise and rehabilitation programs are based on the idea that the spine is meant to flex. A healthy spine is able to move fluidly through a full range of motion, but the spine is not supposed to be extremely flexible. The spine is your body's center of stability, and the muscles surrounding your spine are your primary stabilizers. When the spine is braced as you hinge at the hip joints, you strengthen the hips, the hamstrings, the lower and upper back muscles—the entire powerful posterior chain. Movement originates in your pelvis, hips, and hip joints. Your glutes should be used as propelling muscles that help move your body forward.

Foundation training will teach you to move the way your body is meant to move. We are talking about primitive movement patterns. Think of how a

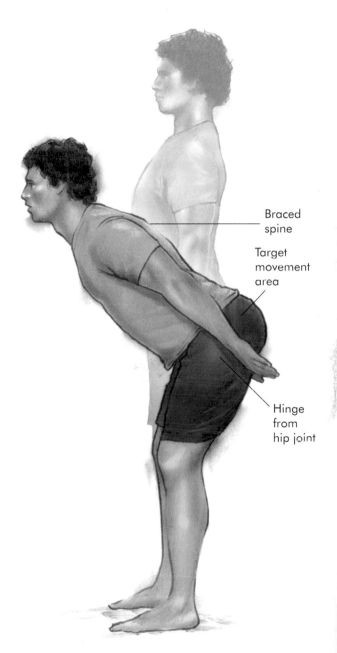

Braced spine

Target movement area

Hinge from hip joint

Extended Spine

four-legged animal moves. It pushes off from its hind legs. An animal digs what would be its back heels into the ground to propel itself forward. The spine stays rigid, and movement originates in the hips and hamstrings. If an animal tried to move from its belly, it would end up curled in a ball. Our bodies evolved to be upright, but the joint lines are still that of four-legged animals.

> Even the professional athletes we train say that they are performing with significantly more power and confidence.

If you watch a young child squat to the ground, the butt sticks out, the back stays completely straight, and the head stays up. This is a perfect anatomical movement pattern.

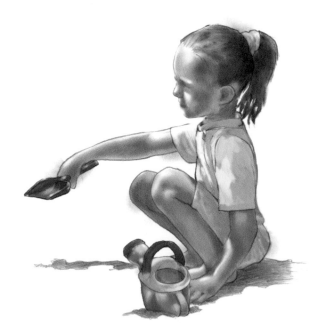

Our aim is to get you to move along the joint lines through which your body is meant to move. All of our exercises teach integrated movement. You will learn to use your hamstrings and glutes as propelling muscles that push you forward.

We call our program Foundation training for a reason. Proper movement is the basis for anything physical you want to do—running, dancing, lifting weights, biking, golfing, playing tennis, or swimming. Once your bad movement patterns are a thing of the past, you will find that taking up any sport or form of exercise becomes easier. Not only will you be able to learn a new activity quickly, but you will be able to reach a higher level of proficiency in that activity than you would have before you fixed your movement patterns. Foundation training creates a strong center or base from which you can branch out. Even the professional athletes we train say that they are performing with significantly more power and confidence.

FOUNDATIONFIRST

Matthew McConaughey, actor

I thought my lower back would be my Achilles' heel forever. Foundation training took that thought out of the equation. I feel strong and flexible, and my posture is better than it has ever been. This stuff is just plain good for you.

Your lower spine is meant to be stable, and Foundation exercises initially teach and then reinforce that stability. By first correcting poor movement patterns, Foundation trains you to use your most powerful muscles properly, creating lasting power and flexibility throughout the most important areas of your body. The proper balance of many small muscles is essential for a healthy spine, free movement, and a full range of motion.

If you are not moving properly, your spine is not in its natural curve and the muscles in your butt cannot contract properly. When the butt muscles can't contract, the spine is not braced, the hamstrings are not long, the quads at the front of your thighs are working too hard, and you place too much

> Foundation trains you to use your most powerful muscles properly, creating lasting power and flexibility throughout the most important areas of your body.

pressure on your knees. If your spine is flexed, all of your weight is pitched forward onto much weaker joints of the body instead of on the big, strong hip muscles. When the hip joints are not absorbing the force they are designed to absorb, that stress goes to the knees and spine. Your spine cannot support that much force. It is meant to absorb straight up-and-down forces, not rotation or forward-and-backward forces. If you hinge at the lower spine, a massive amount of pressure is applied to the discs there, creating movement that far exceeds how much that area is supposed to move. Back pain is one of the results.

When you try to loosen up in a yoga or flexibility class or get on a bike or run, you stretch these weak joints further. Instead of stretching the hips and lengthening the hamstrings properly by hinging from the hips with bent knees, you're hinging with straight legs and a rounded spine, accentuating the forces of flexibility onto that weak area.

What Foundation training uniquely does, in the most simplified terms, is strengthen and train the many small muscles of the spine to brace the entire lower

FOUNDATIONFIRST

LEARNING TO MOVE AGAIN

A few years ago, I experienced a brain injury that caused a neurological deficit on the left side of my body, ultimately leading to a massive loss of strength and coordination. The neurological damage and weak muscles shut down my left leg, made running impossible, and caused me to walk with a pronounced limp.

I spent 18 months working with physical therapists, neurologists, chiropractors, and trainers. I wasn't making the gains I felt I should be. I was stuck in the same place, and I was starting to lose faith that I could correct the deficits to be able to walk normally or ever run again. I was so frustrated. A friend recommended I check out the work Eric Goodman was doing.

After only 7 weeks of working with Eric, I was far ahead of anywhere I had been in the previous 18 months of rehabilitation. My walking gait was close to normal.

I know I am an extreme case, but learning to change my movement patterns has caused me to view what I can do physically in a whole new light. I was convinced I would never be able to compete in a triathlon again because of the running, but now I see it in the near future. I still have a lot of work to do, but with Foundation training, I know I can return to the level of athleticism I had before the injury.

BRAD SEAMAN, USA CYCLING LEVEL 2 EXPERT COACH,
BOULDER PERFORMANCE NETWORK

STRETCHING WITH STRAIGHT LEGS

If you stretch with your legs straight, the emphasis of the stretch is on the far ends of the muscles, where they insert into the joints. On the other hand, the angle produced by bending your knees slightly and hinging from your hips creates more stretch in the belly of your hamstrings. Hinging from your hips with an extended back does not stress the vertebrae of your lower spine and your knees in the way that bending over with a flexed back and straight legs does. Your hips are designed to take that pressure. Your knees and fragile lower spine are not.

Some forms of exercise require you to flex your spine. That movement can be fine as long as your exercise program includes other movements that work the posterior chain. It is a question of balance.

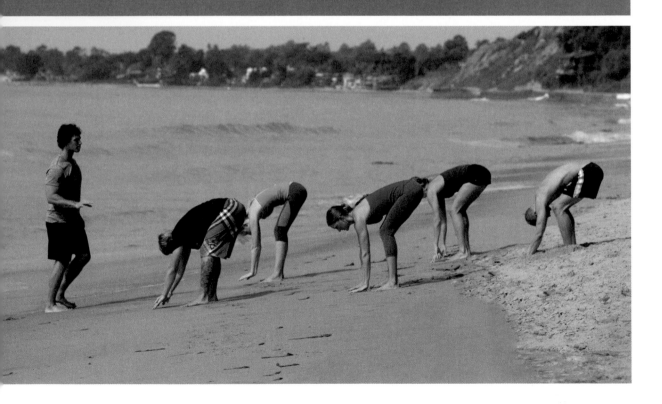

spine while the hips pivot. These muscles are usually used incorrectly. They are made for simple stability and not powerful movement. When you move incorrectly, you are asking these muscles to do a job they are not designed to do. It's like asking a toothpick to do the job of a tree trunk. When these muscles are strong, they have the ability to stabilize the spine while the larger muscles move around them. If your movement originates in the hips and your large posterior muscles, the muscles surrounding the vertebrae are no longer being compressed or overworked. All of that tension, all of that compression, all of that friction is distributed to the hips, glute muscles, and hamstrings, instead of being placed on that tiny spine muscle and that vulnerable disc.

When people with back problems begin to work with a trainer or doctor, they expect a quick fix. They will do the handful of exercises they are given and will go on with their lives when they are feeling better. Those exercises are quickly forgotten. If they do the traditional exercises when needed, they are able to bring themselves to a certain level of comfort. But they never really change their movement patterns beyond the exercises. They never establish a movement or an idea based on the exercises that they can apply to their walking, hiking, cycling, or sitting. We believe that exercise is supposed to change your body. For exercise to be effective, it should be reinforced by everything else you do.

What is new about the Foundation lifestyle is that these exercises are continuously reinforced as your movement patterns begin to change. The stronger you get with the exercises, the more you use them without even thinking about it in your daily life, from the most demanding activity to the least. As soon as the movement pattern establishes itself, it just gets stronger.

A car battery can die and then recharge. As you are driving, the battery

FOUNDATIONFIRST

REFUSING TO BE INACTIVE

I'm a recreational athlete with a few marathons and a 535-mile AIDS bike ride behind me, so I was shocked when I couldn't stand up after working at my computer for a few hours. Suddenly I felt and looked like a fragile 90-year-old woman. Whenever I would get up from a sitting position, pain would radiate from my back to my hip and down my leg. I just couldn't stand up without slowly moving my hips forward. After visits to three doctors, including an osteopath, I learned that my back was locking because of degeneration in my spine. All three doctors told me that I shouldn't run anymore. I had just turned 50, and I refused to accept this verdict. I had already decided to take on a friend's challenge to summit Mount Whitney, the highest mountain in the continental United States. I knew I needed help if I wanted to achieve this dream.

Several years earlier, I had trained successfully with Peter Park. I knew I needed his mojo again. When I called, he told me about the exciting workouts that he had been perfecting with his new partner, Eric Goodman. I was ready for anything.

During just the first workout, I was amazed at what I felt in my body. Different muscles were quivering as I held poses that were similar to but distinctly different from Pilates and yoga. I felt better after just one session, and I was eager for more. During the next 3 months, I worked out with Peter and Eric. It wasn't long before my back pain was gone and I started tackling some runs. Within 6 months, I was able to complete my Mount Whitney challenge, and my body felt great. I had my old self back.

JAN HILL

recharges more and more to the point that it sustains its own energy. The next time you start your car, you won't need a jump start. The same principle applies to Foundation training. The more you do the exercises initially, the more ingrained the movement pattern becomes. When you begin to move this way naturally, you will find that you do not need to do the exercises as often—but most of our clients do them anyway, because the exercises make them feel so good. Foundation training will carry over into every facet of your life, making you vibrant, active, and healthy.

By focusing on your real core, Foundation training will rebalance your body, help you achieve effortless good posture, increase your flexibility, invigorate your movement, and, most important, ensure long-lasting back health.

In this chapter, we have shown you what sets Foundation training apart from every other exercise program. We have explained the philosophy and mechanics behind Foundation training and why the program works so well, even for people who had given up hope.

Now that you know why we had to redefine the core to get long-term results, we want to show you how these unique exercises work to relieve back pain and why they are so successful in preventing its return. To explain why the movements of Foundation training are so effective, we have to consider the anatomical sources of acute and chronic back pain. In the following chapter, The Roots of Back Pain, we will take a close look at what can go wrong.

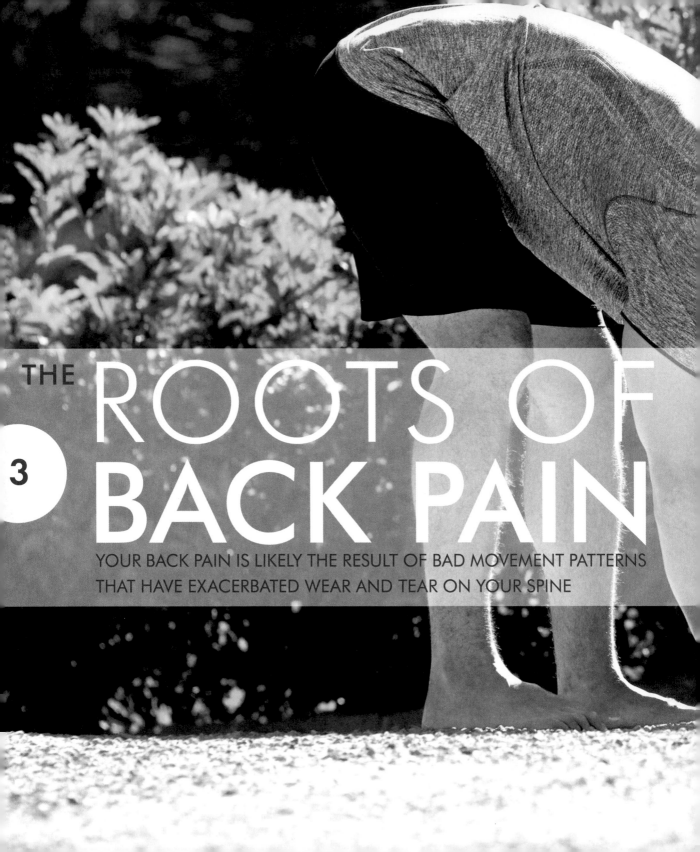

THE ROOTS OF BACK PAIN

3

YOUR BACK PAIN IS LIKELY THE RESULT OF BAD MOVEMENT PATTERNS
THAT HAVE EXACERBATED WEAR AND TEAR ON YOUR SPINE

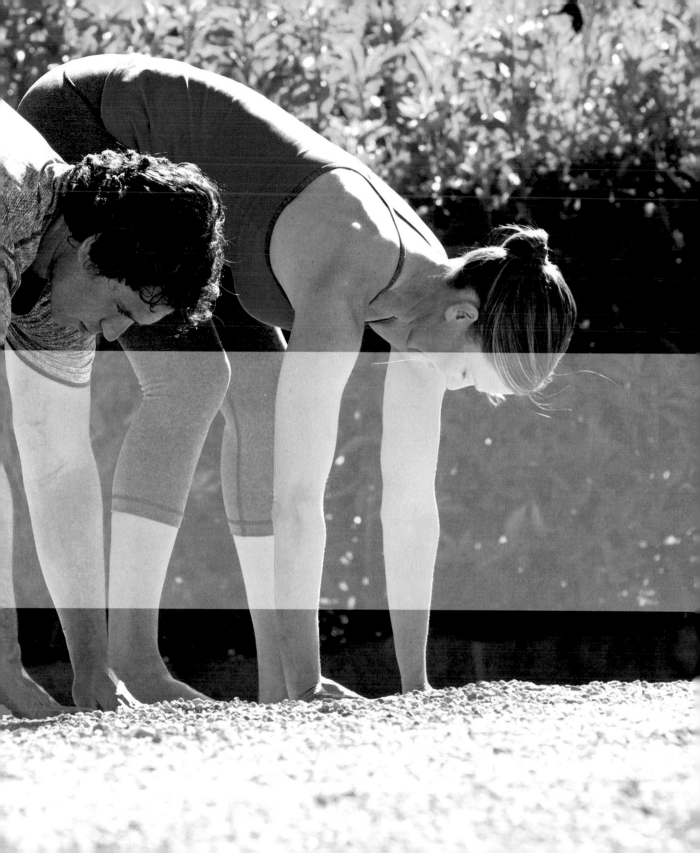

How did your pain begin? Though this question is asked commonly when diagnosing back pain, it tends to yield misleading answers no matter how you look at it. If you assume that the instant you began to feel pain was when your back problem began, you are looking at a symptom. Unless some blunt force trauma or accident happened, your back problem started long before the pain. Your back pain is most likely the result of wear and tear on your spine that has been exacerbated by long-term bad movement patterns. In this chapter, we will look at how various spinal problems result from moving in ways your body is not designed to do.

> Unless some blunt force trauma or accident happened, your back problem started long before the pain.

Pain is a tricky thing. What does your pain feel like? Whether it's dull, sharp, hot, cold, deep, superficial, or just plain achy, it can make life harder. There are types of pain that require more attention than others. Be aware of what your body is telling you. If you have sharp, intense back pain for the first time, you should see a doctor for a diagnosis before treating yourself. Sudden, intense back pain or pain that never goes away can be a symptom of serious illness. When you first experience back pain, there is no better option than to visit a trusted medical practitioner.

Eighty percent of all back pain is acute, severe but short-lived. Acute, subacute, chronic—for many people, these back pain timelines do not offer answers. Guess what? If you have pain in the same area of your body more than a couple of times, you have an issue that needs to be addressed. Chances are the problem will continue to build if the reason it is occurring is not managed properly.

Our goal in this chapter is to look at the anatomical sources of acute and chronic

WARNING SIGNS

Though you can treat most back pain yourself, pain can be a symptom of serious medical problems. If you experience any of the situations or symptoms listed here, make sure to get medical care.

- A recent accident, including a fall or car accident
- Pain so intense that it awakens you when you are sleeping at night
- Fever higher than 100 degrees, chills, sweats, or other signs of infection
- Unexplained weight loss
- Difficulty with bowel or bladder control
- Pain radiating down one or both legs below the knee
- Difficulty walking, raising or lowering your foot at the ankle, or raising your big toe upward
- Inability to walk on your heels or stand on your toes
- Throbbing in your abdomen

If you have a history of cancer, osteoporosis, steroid use, or drug or alcohol abuse, it is important that you see a doctor the first time you experience back pain. If your back pain persists for more than a few days without some alleviation, you should consider further evaluation.

back pain by giving you a brief overview of the spine and its potential problems. Armed with an atlas of spinal anatomy, you will be able to envision the various parts of your back and understand why your back is vulnerable and what goes wrong physically to create pain.

THE SPINE

Your spine is a powerful support structure that enables you to stand upright, gives your body shape, and houses nerves that link your brain to the rest of your body. Your spine is composed of the vertebrae and discs of the spinal column, the spinal cord and nerve roots, and the muscles and ligaments that support the bones of the spinal column. These components work together to hold your body erect and protect your spinal cord.

> Your spine is a powerful support structure that enables you to stand upright, gives your body shape, and houses nerves that link your brain to the rest of your body.

There are 24 vertebrae and two separate bones stacked on top of each other to provide a flexible support structure that protects the spinal cord from injury. More than 70 small facet joints between the vertebrae allow the spine to move. The vertebrae are separated by dense gelatinous discs, which serve as cushions—usually. Hundreds of small ligaments and muscles attached to the back of the spine provide power for movement and support.

THE HARDWARE OF THE SPINAL COLUMN

The sacrum attaches the spine to the pelvis. The five lumbar vertebrae of the lower back (L1–5) are the seat of most back pain. The lumbar spine should not support the weight of the upper body but should brace the back in order for the glutes to function in absorbing that weight. However, if you do not hinge from the hip, your lower back is involved in bending, extending, and rotating at the waist and has to support the weight of the upper body. Moving in this way puts a great strain on this region of your back, which is already heavily engaged in stabilizing the spine. Foundation training is designed to teach you to move with your spine in its natural curve to reduce the stress on your lower back.

THE CURVES OF YOUR SPINE

The spinal column has three sections that create three natural curves in your back at the neck, rib cage, and lower back.

There are inward curves at the neck and

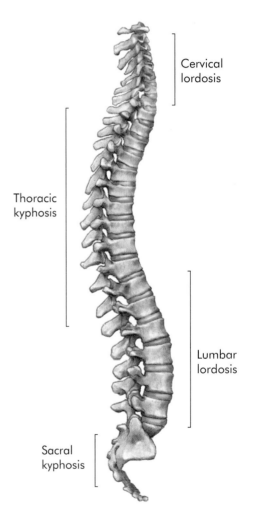

Cervical lordosis

Thoracic kyphosis

Lumbar lordosis

Sacral kyphosis

Spinal Column

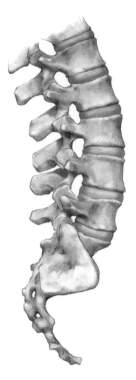

The Trouble Zone: Lumbar Spine

lower back (lordosis) and an outward curve at the chest level (kyphosis). As you can see in the illustration above, the lower spine has a small forward curve. The lordotic curve of the lumbar spine is responsible for the proper movement of the glutes and hips. Without this curve, the butt muscles are unable to contract properly.

Internal rotation and improper hinging work against the natural curve of your spine, throwing your back out of alignment. Flattening your lower back by tipping your pelvis forward is not good for the stability of your spine. If you flatten the lordotic curve of the lower back, known as hypolordosis, your glutes cannot be

FOUNDATIONFIRST

ENDING THE CYCLE OF INJURY

Peter and Eric have created the perfect storm, bringing together evidence-based science and functional training that is second to none. Their approach to building a solid foundation is my prescription for everyone from the top athletes in the world to their mothers! Movement is life. Life is movement. And if you are limited in how you move against the constant forces of gravity, it is only a matter of time until you are injured. I know this to be true as I have experienced this roller coaster as a competitive athlete. Not until I retrained my movement patterns did the cycle of injury after injury end.

It really is a thing of beauty to see such a brilliant melding of creativity and sports science built into a practical, low-tech program that focuses on posture, core, and fundamental movement patterns designed first and foremost to provide athletes with a solid foundation to apply to their chosen sport. I'll never forget what Derek Fisher said to Peter and Eric about why he chose to work with them: "I did not hire you to make me a better basketball player; I hired you to make me a better athlete." True, true.

TIM BROWN, DC, FOUNDER OF INTELLISKIN

activated fully, and your lower back has to absorb more pressure and weight than it is designed to do, resulting in back pain.

THE FORTRESS

The stacked vertebrae create a canal that protects the spinal cord, which carries messages from your brain to your muscles and vice versa. The spinal cord runs from the base of your brain to about two-thirds down your back. At the lumbar level, a bunch of nerve roots, called the cauda equina, or horse's tail, continues. The spine ends just after the cauda equina, at a spot called the filum terminale. This gap in the lower spinal cord is what allows for lumbar punctures, epidurals, and other procedures to occur without directly affecting the cord.

Forty-eight nerves branch out from the spinal cord through openings in the vertebrae. At each vertebra, a pair of nerve roots supplies neural impulses to a particular part of the body. The nerve roots of the lumbar spine provide sensations and stimulate the muscles of the lower back and lower extremities.

Small facet joints located between vertebrae allow your spine to move. Each vertebra has four facet joints: a pair that faces upward and another that faces

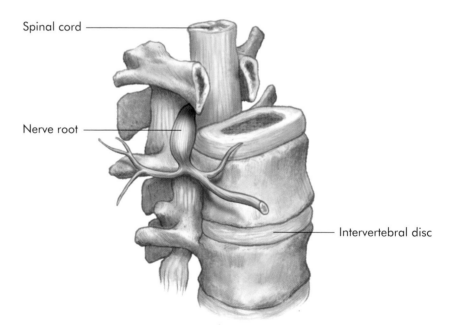

Nerves of the Spine

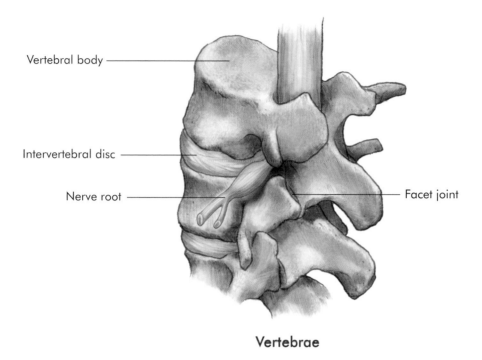

Vertebral body

Intervertebral disc

Nerve root

Facet joint

Vertebrae

downward. The facet joints interlock with the adjacent vertebrae to provide stability to the spine.

The vertebrae are separated by flat, round discs that are about ½ inch thick. They have a tough outer coating that connects to the vertebrae, and their center is a soft gel. The discs act as shock absorbers, preventing the vertebrae from banging or rubbing against each other.

We are including an illustration of the layers of back muscles and ligaments (see page 43) because we want you to have a sense of the intricate network required to keep your spine stable and flexible at the same time.

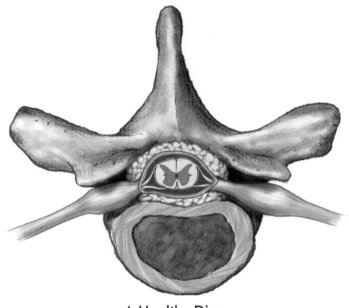

A Healthy Disc

Hundred of ligaments, which attach bones to bones, connect the vertebrae. It takes hundreds of muscles in your back to control movement. Gravity, wear and tear, bad movement patterns, and computer syndrome take their toll on your spine, but you can slow down the degenerative process with Foundation training.

BACK ISSUES

Lower-back pain can be triggered by a number of factors, often in combination. Overuse, muscle strain, and trauma to muscles, ligaments, bones, and discs make the back vulnerable to injury and reinjury. If you perform the same motion over and over without a properly braced spine, you can develop repetitive back strain and injure your discs and vertebrae. Bending, lifting, running, reaching, and sitting all involve your back muscles. If you are not moving properly, your spine, particularly your lumbar spine, will be subjected to significant wear and tear.

In the event that you do strain muscles, ligaments, facet joints, or sacroiliac joints (the joints between the sacrum and the iliac bone of the pelvis), you might in turn change the way you move to avoid the pain, exaggerating bad movement patterns even further. We have all seen people walking along with one hip hitched up, favoring one side of their body.

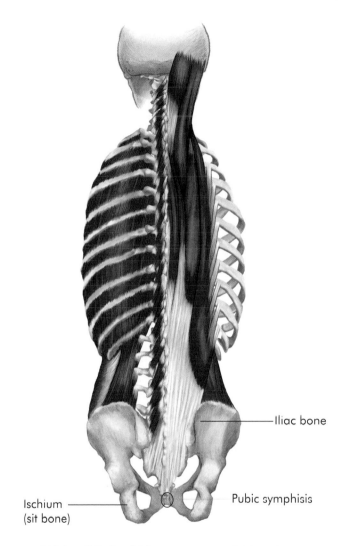

Web of Spinal Ligaments and Muscles

Iliac bone

Pubic symphisis

Ischium
(sit bone)

Compensating this way causes you to strain other muscles that are not designed to move the way you are using them, setting off a vicious cycle of injury and pain.

Rather than taxing muscles that are not meant to work so hard, you will learn to move in a way that allows the posterior chain to do its job with integrated, powerful movement.

The truth is, by the time most of us reach our forties, we experience discomfort in our lower backs after years of moving badly, stressing the soft tissues of this region mechanically. Avoiding this type of mechanical stress is what Foundation training is all about. Rather than taxing muscles that are not meant to work so hard, you will learn to move in a way that allows the posterior chain to do its job with integrated, powerful movement.

MUSCLE SPASMS

A back spasm—it feels like a charley horse in your calf—is a powerful involuntary contraction in response to an injury or oxygen deficiency. The spasm is so strong that it sometimes prevents you from moving. The spasm is a response that protects an injury by immobilizing you, preventing you from aggravating the injury.

A back spasm is a sign that you have injured something else. A torn ligament, tendon, or severe muscle damage; a ruptured disc pressing on a nerve; an infection; and an irritated joint could all trigger a muscle spasm. In the next chapter, you will learn about the iliopsoas group of muscles that runs from several lower-back vertebrae through the pelvis to the inner thigh. This group of muscles often spasms when a ligament or disc in the lower spine is damaged, resulting in hip and back pain.

FOUNDATIONFIRST

Jeff Bridges, actor

My back likes to let me know when it's pissed at me. When it does, life can become a bit more challenging. Foundation exercises have been a great addition to my exercise routine. I really notice a change in how I move. My back doesn't just feel better, it feels strong. That is a big deal. These exercises let you move with some real confidence. Everybody with a bad back should do these exercises.

DISC ISSUES

Chronic back problems are usually not muscular but instead originate from pressure on the nerve roots that leave the spinal column. This compression is sometimes caused by a bulging disc. By the time you are 40, the gel within your discs has begun to dehydrate and shrink, and the exterior cartilage can crack, irritating the

A back spasm is a sign that you have injured something else.

surrounding nerves and muscles. Small tears to the outer part of the disc can produce a full spectrum of pain response, from no pain to disabling chronic pain. We cannot explain why the effects of disc tears vary so much from person to person.

If a disc is worn or injured, the gel at its center may squeeze through the outer ring. A herniated or ruptured disc can squeeze from between two vertebrae into the spinal canal or into the opening from which the nerves exit the vertebrae. The nerve becomes directly irritated. When a herniated disc bulges toward the spinal canal, the pressure on the spinal nerves causes pain. This occurs most frequently with the discs of the fourth and fifth vertebrae of the lower back.

When a nerve is directly impinged upon, you may experience a sharp pain at the site of the pressure, sometimes accompanied by numbness in the area of the leg that the affected nerve supplies, or you may feel radiating pain along the nerve's pathway. Since the nervous system communicates with your muscles by electrical

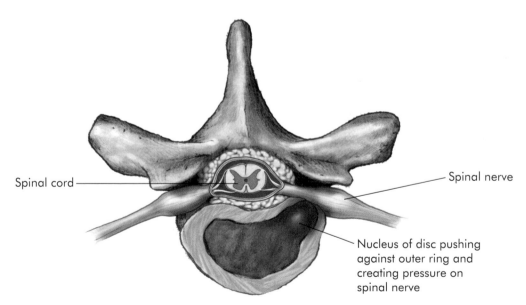

Spinal cord

Spinal nerve

Nucleus of disc pushing against outer ring and creating pressure on spinal nerve

Cross-Section View of Herniated Lumbar Disc

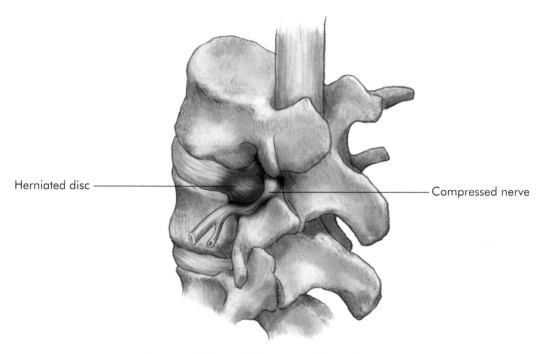

Herniated disc ——————————————   —— Compressed nerve

Lateral View of Herniated Lumbar Disc

impulses, a ruptured disc can disrupt or block this communication, which results in weakened muscles. If the weakness is severe, it could indicate a significant problem. When you experience acute muscle weakness, you should definitely see a doctor.

The nerves of the lower back control the hips, legs, and feet. Each of the nerve roots sends its impulses on a specific pathway. A herniated disc in the lower back can put pressure on a nerve root that leads to the leg and foot, causing pain to radiate to the buttock and down the leg, which is called referred pain. You do not necessarily have pain at the site of the ruptured disc.

The sciatic nerve, the longest and widest nerve in the body, runs from the lower

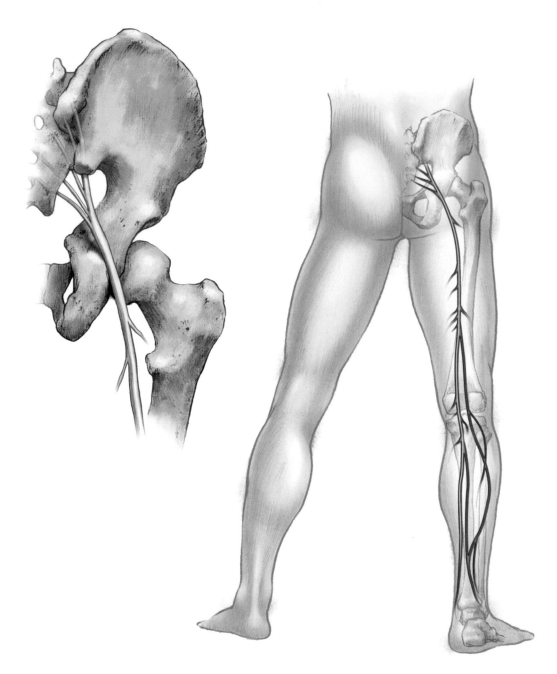

Sciatic Nerve

back through the butt and down the back of each leg to the foot. The term *sciatica* is often used to describe pain down the back of the leg. Sciatica is not a diagnosis. Sciatica is a symptom of another medical problem rather than a condition in and of itself. Pain down the back of the leg can be caused by many things. A ruptured disc or bone

FOUNDATIONFIRST

REHABILITATION WITH FOUNDATION TRAINING

I had recently undergone a successful surgery to repair a herniated disc. Months of traditional physical therapy had not improved my recovery. I was afraid of incurring another injury and avoided important events and simple activities. I found my way to Foundation training. I learned that I did not have to change my life or my expectations to accommodate pain.

I was thrilled by the progress I made in just a few short weeks. My success is owed to the program's brilliant simplicity. I find myself practicing the exercises throughout the day and challenging my ability with ease. I am looking forward to the possibility of being in the best physical condition of my life.

I have been so eager to spread the word about Foundation training that I invite my family and friends to join my one-on-one sessions. From my 11-year-old son, who swims competitively, to my parents, who want to enjoy gardening and playing with their young grandchildren, we have found a new movement plan that will take us through each of our lifetimes. This is a great bodywork for all ages and abilities—something you can do anytime, anywhere. And the more you do it, the better it feels. The Foundation program offers so much more than pain relief. It is the beginning of a new way of thinking about fitness. The Foundation offers us all the best type of health insurance—gain without pain!

ALEX DAUGHERTY, WIFE AND MOTHER OF TWO YOUNG CHILDREN

spur could be putting pressure on the nerve root that leads to the sciatic nerve.

Although herniated discs are found in many people over age 20, only a small percentage of herniated discs produce symptoms of nerve impingement.

DEGENERATIVE DISC DISEASE

Though degenerative disc disease sounds serious, the condition is almost universal. Discs begin to degenerate by the time most of us reach our twenties. By the age of 30, most people have mild to moderate disc degeneration in one or more discs in the lower back or neck. Discs lose moisture and volume as they age. Their thickness and circumference decrease, reducing the distance between vertebrae. The shrinking of that cushion makes the spine more vulnerable. The reduced distance between vertebrae can cause the bones to rub against each other.

Inflammation and nerve root involvement can occur even without a rupture in the disc, because the vertebrae themselves can compress a nerve root. Moving badly or slouching for hours is tough on your vertebrae, especially when your discs provide less of a cushion. There is a reason discs tend to degenerate in the neck and lower back. Poor posture, a sedentary lifestyle, and improper movement contribute to the degeneration of discs in those regions.

As disc dehydration progresses with age and the height and mass of the discs shrink, the vertebrae come closer together, making a person slightly shorter each year. Moving with a braced spine and good posture will go a long way toward preserving your height.

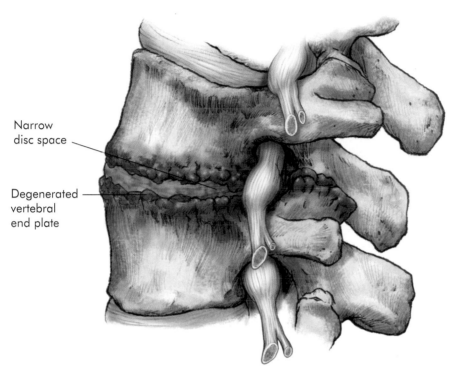

Narrow
disc space

Degenerated
vertebral
end plate

Degenerative Disc Disease

OSTEOARTHRITIS

Degeneration of the joints also develops with age. Arthritis in the spine occurs when the cartilage in the aligning facet joints of the spine erodes as a result of wear and tear, injury, or misuse. The facet joints thicken and harden with age, which can create painful friction. The overgrowth of bone can form bone spurs that can press on nerve roots. Once again, proper movement will take stress and pressure off the joints in your spine, which can help you avoid developing this condition or at least keep it from progressing.

FOUNDATION FIRST

Kelly Slater, world championship surfer

I am somewhat new to Foundation training, but I can already feel what this work is capable of. My back has always been an issue, and I know Foundation will get me where I need to be to win my 10th world title.*

*Kelly went on to win his 10th world title in 2010.

If you have arthritis in your hips or knees, you might compensate for the pain in the way you move and walk. That alteration in your movement patterns can strain your muscles and throw your back out of alignment, which further contributes to your pain.

SPINAL STENOSIS

Spinal disc degeneration in combination with arthritis in the joints of the lower back can lead to a narrowing of the space around the spinal cord. Spinal stenosis may cause pain that radiates down both legs after standing or walking for an extended period.

Depending on what nerves are affected, stenosis can cause pain or numbness in your neck, shoulders, arms, and legs. You can experience weakness or lose sensation in your extremities as well. This condition should be monitored by a doctor.

SPONDYLOLYSIS AND SPONDYLOLISTHESIS

Spondylolysis is a defect in the connection between vertebrae; specifically, a thin piece of bone that connects the upper and lower segments of facet joints. The defect leads to small stress fractures that weaken the vertebrae.

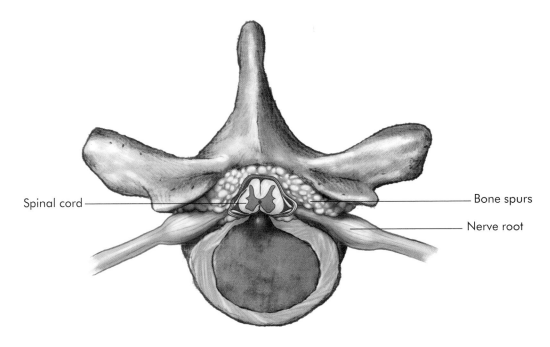

Spinal cord

Bone spurs

Nerve root

Spinal Stenosis

If the facet joints become very weak because of the degeneration of normally stabilizing structures, a vertebra can slip out of place, moving forward or back in alignment from the spinal column. The forward-moving condition is known as spondylolisthesis.

People born with thin vertebrae are at higher risk for developing spondylolysis. Repetitive trauma can also contribute. Spondylolysis is a common cause of lower-back pain in people under age 26, particularly athletes who put a lot of stress on their backs or hyperextend or overstretch their spines constantly. The sports that appear to be most damaging are gymnastics, basketball, football, and weight lifting, but any high-impact activity can aggravate the condition.

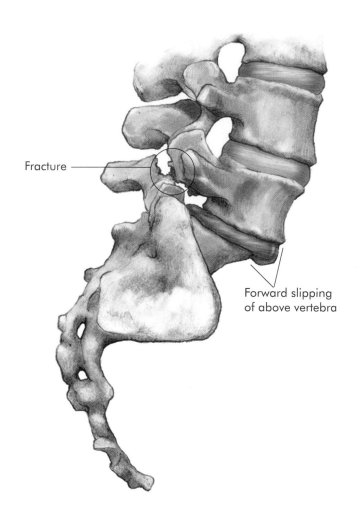

Fracture

Forward slipping
of above vertebra

Spondylolisthesis

PREGNANCY AND BACK PAIN

Weight gain during pregnancy puts extra stress on the spine. Additionally, as a woman progresses through pregnancy, her uterus grows and her stomach muscles become overstretched and cannot handle the entire weight of the uterus. The spine and back muscles have to work harder to carry the weight.

Additionally, a woman's center of gravity shifts forward when she is pregnant. You've probably observed that pregnant women move differently; those movement patterns may not be good for the back. It's common for women to compensate to maintain balance, and this can strain the muscles of the lower back.

Complicating matters further, hormones relax the muscles, ligaments, and joints in a woman's pelvis to prepare for giving birth. The loose joints that attach the pelvis to the spine weaken the support the back usually gets.

The problems don't end with childbirth. New mothers typically get little rest, and they carry around not only the baby but also all the equipment that comes with the territory. It's a perfect storm for a back injury.

It makes sense to prepare your body for carrying your baby by incorporating Foundation training into your exercise program *before* you get pregnant. A strong spine will help you avoid back pain during pregnancy.

Once you are pregnant, you should discuss these exercises with your obstetrician and follow his or her recommendations. As a general rule, we suggest that you avoid the floor work during pregnancy, but doing the standing Foundation exercises will help your pelvis stay strong and your pelvic muscles relax as you go through the stages of pregnancy. Your recuperation will be easier as well if your pelvic muscles are well toned.

THE BIG PICTURE

There are many other causes of back pain, including weakening of the vertebrae resulting from osteoporosis, which is often seen in women over 50. What we've discussed here is just an overview of some of the most common types of back pain; we'll refrain from getting into esoteric and serious conditions. Suffice it to say that the vast majority of people who consult with a doctor about lower-back pain never get a concrete diagnosis. The cause of their pain cannot be identified. This brings us back to an important point we made earlier: Foundation training is not designed to treat a condition. Instead, it gets to the root of the pain by correcting the mechanical problems that lead to imbalance and weakness that cause stress and friction in the spine. Herniated discs, degenerative disc disease, osteoarthritis, spinal stenosis, and degenerative

> The vast majority of people who consult with a doctor about lower-back pain never get a concrete diagnosis.

joint disease all have one thing in common: bad movement patterns. Foundation training will correct them.

In the next chapter, The Anatomy of Foundation Movement, we will show you how correcting the way you move works so effectively to alleviate pain with long-term results.

FOUNDATIONFIRST

BACK ON THE COURT WITH POWER

Derek Fisher told me about Eric and Foundation training toward the end of the 2010 Championship season. I was skeptical and coming from a place with a lot of frustration because of my back injury. But I figure if Fish says something is worth trying, it's probably true, so I set up an appointment.

   The first day was rough. I mean, I was just shaking. I think that's kind of the idea at first—to show strong athletes how weak they are in the most important areas. Within a couple of sessions, I was able to really feel my back muscles working. In fact, it was like the deep muscles in my back had been turned on. I don't want to say I had all that much hope at first, but I could tell this was creating some change. My goal is to play in the NBA as long as I can and to always be an asset to the team. I tried everything to get past my back injury. I feel powerful right now. Foundation training has given me legitimate hope.

LUKE WALTON, LA LAKER

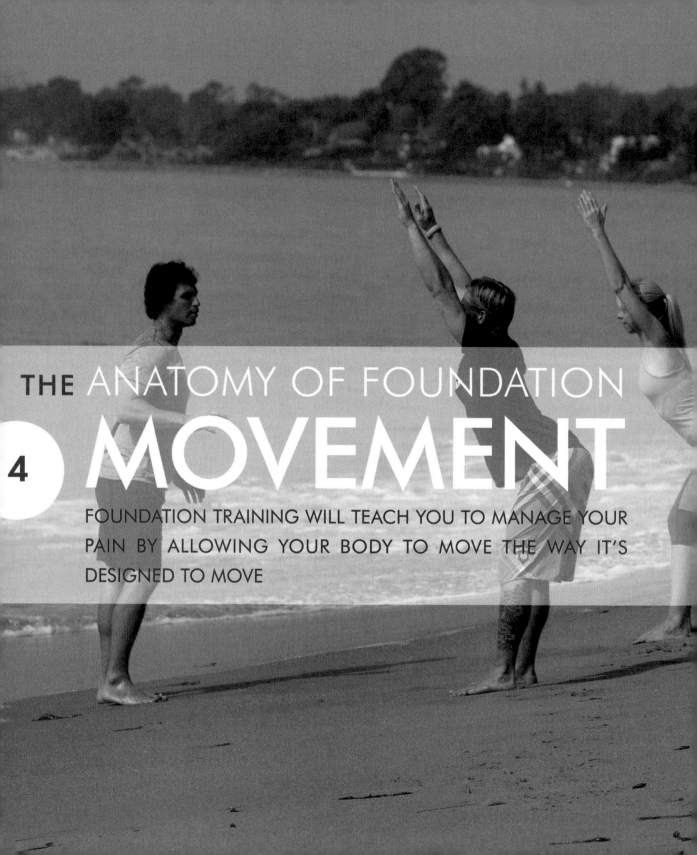

THE ANATOMY OF FOUNDATION

4

MOVEMENT

FOUNDATION TRAINING WILL TEACH YOU TO MANAGE YOUR PAIN BY ALLOWING YOUR BODY TO MOVE THE WAY IT'S DESIGNED TO MOVE

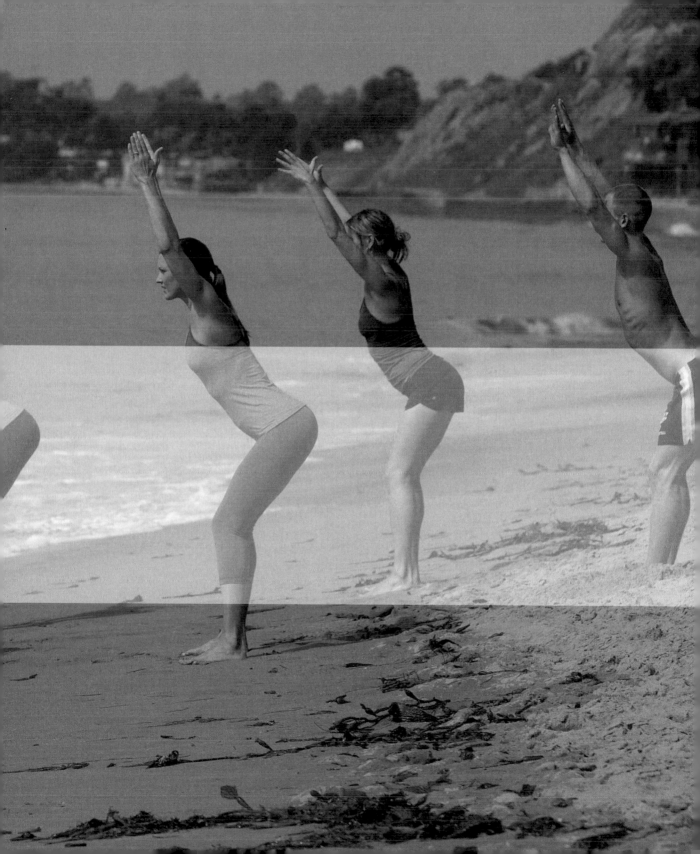

f you've suffered from back pain for any significant amount of time, you've probably absorbed an endless amount of information about the injuries and conditions that cause it, but as you also know well, no one provides a simple plan of action that works for long-lasting pain relief.

Foundation training will teach you to manage your pain without drugs or surgery by allowing your body to move the way it is designed to move. Degeneration in your spine is a result of too much friction, pressure, and abrasion. Aside from producing wear and tear on your vertebrae and discs, the pressure and friction that faulty movement patterns produce can stimulate your spine to lay down calcium, which builds up, changes your movement, and can impinge on your nerves. Foundation training minimizes the progression of degeneration by reducing the pressure on your spine. Degeneration occurs where the most force happens. When we shift the pressure from the injured area to the larger muscles of the posterior chain, there is no longer significant friction. To put it simply, Foundation training braces the injured areas while shifting the movement to the powerful muscles designed to do the job, allowing you to manage your injuries with movement as opposed to managing injuries because of improper movement.

An x-ray of Eric's spine today would show that his degeneration is just as bad, if not worse, than it was when his back problems were originally diagnosed. The degeneration will not go away, and his discs are still compressed. The difference is this: It does not hurt anymore. He is stronger, more flexible, and in better shape than he has ever been in his life. In the same vein, by changing his movement patterns, Peter no longer suffers after a long run, demanding ride, or tough workout. Moving differently is saving his joints.

Our own experiences and those of all of our clients have made it clear that Foundation training works. If you can learn to move your body in the right way, to hinge and pivot properly, to strengthen your hips and your entire body, and to use your butt muscles and hamstrings properly to take pressure away from the front of your body and your spine, you can control your chronic injuries. Normally, you would be going to doctors and physical therapists, taking over-the-counter or prescription painkillers, and icing yourself down in order to manage your symptoms.

Once you incorporate the movements of Foundation training into your life, however, the symptoms you have been struggling with will begin to go away. Foundation training will alleviate your pain and give you a tool you can always use to deal with current pain and prevent future pain.

> Foundation training will alleviate your pain and give you a tool you can always use to deal with current pain and prevent future pain.

Now that you've taken our crash course in the anatomy of the spine, we can demonstrate how the movements of Foundation training work. It all starts with the hinge.

THE HINGE: THE FOUNDATION OF PROPER MOVEMENT

A healthy spine moves fluidly through a full range of motion at each movable segment, but the spine is not supposed to be extremely flexible. Your hips, shoulders,

FOUNDATIONFIRST

FLUID, EXPLOSIVE MOVEMENT ON THE COURT AGAIN

Foundation has changed the way I approach my professional tennis career. Eric Goodman's unique Foundation exercises and the principles of movement behind them have helped me overcome my injuries and have lifted my performance on the court as I embark on the next part of my career. From the time I turned pro at 18 at Wimbledon in 1999 to 2010, I had a number of injuries, surgery, and 3 years of intense rehabilitation. My life changed when I started working with Peter and Eric.

I was within the top 100 on the Women's Tennis Association Tour during the first 5 years of my career. I had made history when I played from qualifying to the semifinals at Wimbledon in '99. John McEnroe was the only other player to have accomplished the same feat at the same age. I put everything into my tennis on the court. I was known for my strong first serve in the 120s and my powerful second serve at 105 to 115 mph. Off the court, I was training, running, lifting weights, stretching. Every body part was injured during my first 5 years of professional tennis. There is an iconic photo of me in the ESPN files. I am just off the practice court at age 18, with an ice bag on my right shoulder and ice strapped to both knees and my thigh. Trainers and coaches told me to just keep lifting, running, and stretching and it would all work out.

In October 2002, I reached my highest ranking of 18. I reached the finals of Linz, a WTA event at the end of the season, where I faced Justine Henin. The only problem was that I had pulled my adductor in my upper left leg, and I had a SI joint injury in my lower back. It was a sold-out crowd of 5,000 people. I had to play. The trainers taped me like a mummy. I played and lost. When the match was over, I couldn't move to my left, and my arm felt like knees, and ankles are built to hinge; your back is not. For your spine to remain stable, the flexibility at the level of the vertebrae should be minimal.

Flexibility and forward bending should come from gross joint movements at the hips and not from the spine. This concept and change in movement patterns form

a dead weight. I flew home with a beautiful crystal runner-up trophy and a beat-up body. No one had an answer for me, so I kept stretching, icing, lifting, and running.

At Wimbledon the next year, I felt an electric shock go down my arm in the second round. I couldn't lift my arm to serve. I had torn my labrum. Since strengthening protocols didn't work, I had surgery on my right shoulder. My right arm was as important to me as a pitching arm is to a baseball pitcher. After an intensive rehab, I couldn't get fluid motion in my shoulder. I resisted having another surgery and began a prolonged pitcher rehab program that went on for 3 years. In 2009, I picked up an injury to my foot, and the adductor continued to bother me.

Just this year I began training with Peter Park, and he introduced me to Eric Goodman and Foundation training. Everything in my tennis life changed. My movements to my forehand are more fluid. My running for short balls is quicker. I feel taller. I am able to serve in the 120s again, but the most significant change is my second serve, which is now a powerful weapon in a match. I wake up in the morning loose—without stiffness in my body. My lower back hasn't hurt since I began the Foundation stretches, and my hips, which have always been tight, have opened up. I go on the court ready to play. I feel more fluid in the game. I notice that my first hit is big, and my legs are long and loose and ready to run for balls. My shoulder doesn't stiffen up in matches or off-court training. Everything flows.

Foundation is helping me have a second career, stay injury free, and exhibit explosive motion on the tennis court. Foundation has removed all of my physical pain. During an examination this fall, my doctor said my shoulders were strong and perfectly aligned for the first time. Foundation has helped me gain this amazing achievement.

ALEXANDRA STEVENSON, PRO TENNIS PLAYER

Flexibility and forward bending should come from gross joint movements at the hips and not from the spine.

the core of Foundation movement. Bending from the waist distorts the natural curves of the spinal column. Some vertebrae are hyper-flexed (overextended), while others are hypoflexed (reduced mobility).

The S-shape of the spinal column should be retained while bending forward, as shown in the illustration below. To avoid injury and brace your spine properly, you need to extend your back in a straight line from your butt to your neck and bend from your hip joint. We use the term "the hinge" with all our clients. It is the basic movement in Foundation training.

Bending this way removes pressure from the discs and places it on the muscles surrounding the vertebrae, which then form a brace for the spine.

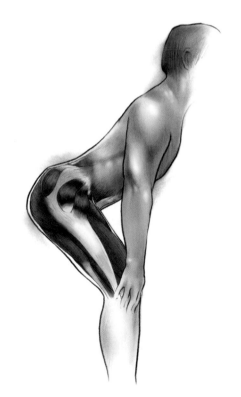

Extended Back, Hinging from the Hips

That is where the new core comes into play. When you correct your movement patterns, all of the tension, compression, and friction go to the hips and posterior chain instead of the tiny spinal muscles. So that you understand what you're supposed to be activating in Foundation training—where movement should come from—let's take a closer look at the powerful muscles that attach directly to the spine or pelvis.

THE STABILIZERS

Of the hundreds of muscles of the spinal column, Foundation training is concerned with three, which are responsible for bracing the spine in extension: the multifidi, erector spinae, and quadratus lumborum. These are the muscles that become over-worked when your movement patterns stress your spine.

Bad posture and movement place these muscles under great strain in their efforts to support your spine.

> Once your back muscles are stronger, your spine will relax, your hamstrings will lengthen, and your glutes will function more powerfully.

Once your back muscles are stronger, your spine will relax, your hamstrings will lengthen, your glutes will function more powerfully, and you will naturally open up. The multifidi, erector spinae, and quadratus lumborum, along with the rotators and interspinales (short

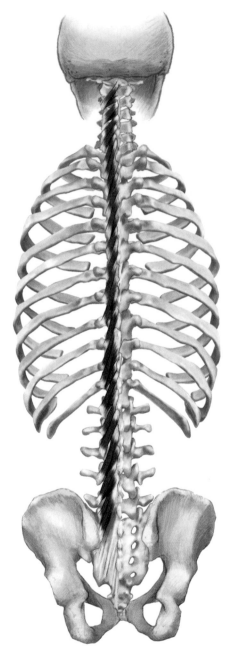

Multifidi

muscular fasciculi between contiguous vertebrae), will hold your spine in extension and enable you to move properly. By removing pressure from the discs and placing it on the muscles that surround the vertebrae, you will reduce pain.

MULTIFIDI

The multifidi are very small muscles that until recently were not considered important to back health. These muscles are deep in the spine. They fill the groove on either side of the vertebrae and span three joints each, providing a scaffolding for the spinal column. They have a unique design that makes the spine stable and keeps you upright. As tiny as they are, they are actually the strongest muscles in the back. The multifidi anticipate motion and stabilize the spine before movement occurs.

They are made up of short, stiff muscles fibers packed inside a casing. This structure gives them extra strength for support. The multifidi take pressure off vertebral discs and distribute body weight evenly.

Recent research has found that back pain patients have a reduced ability to recruit the multifidi to maintain a neutral spine position. In cases of lower-back pain, anticipatory contractions in these muscles have been shown to be delayed or absent. Foundation training corrects these dysfunctions by taking undue stress off the multifidi.

ERECTOR SPINAE

This bundle of muscles and tendons, located in a groove on either side of the vertebral column, is responsible for extension, lateral bending, and

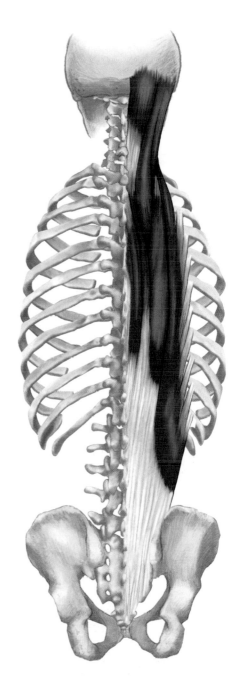

Erector Spinae

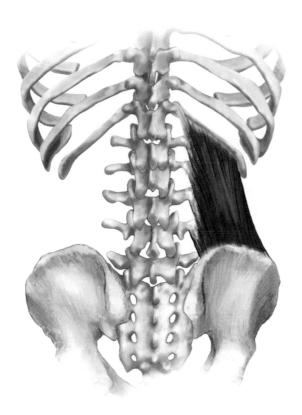

Quadratus Lumborum

rotation. The muscle group starts at the crest at the center of the sacrum and divides into three columns at the small of the back. They have a key role in supporting good posture.

QUADRATUS LUMBORUM

This muscle, located on each side of the body, stabilizes the pelvis and lumbar spine. The muscle is responsible for right and left bending and rotation. Since many of us sit for 90 percent of the day, the quadratus lumborum becomes short, tight, and overused, because each side is constantly working to keep you erect when you sit without lower-back support.

If you habitually cross your legs, your quadratus lumborum will be engaged. When you cross your right leg over your left, you will lean slightly to the left, and your right quadratus lumborum must work hard to keep your upper body erect.

ILIOPSOAS

The iliacus and psoas muscles work together for hip flexion. The iliacus muscle lines the internal border of the pelvis—specifically, the iliac crest, which looks like a wing. The iliacus muscle functions as a secondary hip flexor in combination with the psoas. The iliacus primarily provides pelvic and hip stability, and the psoas is more involved with hip flexion. Tight iliopsoas flexors are not the source of back

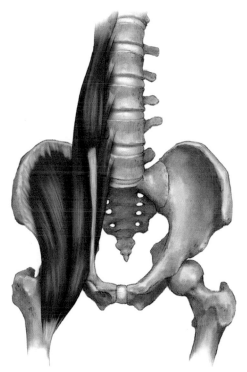

Iliacus and Psoas Muscles

pain but are instead a symptom of a weak spine. You will not get lasting pain relief or significant change from stretching, massaging, or treating the iliopsoas in other ways without strengthening the back extension muscles.

The iliacus is primarily responsible for stabilizing the pelvis and hip joint. When the iliacus is strong and able to contract normally, there is a relaxed pelvic expansion during a squat. If the iliacus spasms during a squat, excessive pressure is put on the knees. If you have a weak iliacus muscle, you will not be able to squat without pressing your knees to the outside of your hips. Since you will find it difficult to shift your hips back over your heels as you stand, the weight will shift away from your glutes to the far weaker quadriceps and knee joints in the front of your leg.

The psoas, an important hip flexor, is often involved in chronic back pain. This muscle attaches the hip to the upper lumbar spine and will either pull the spine down or the hip up when flexing. If your spine is powerful, it will stay straight and strong while you raise your hip. If your spine is weak, you will end up bending both the hip and spine and will ultimately have a great deal of pain. Psoas tightness is often considered responsible for back pain, and the psoas is treated to relieve back pain instead of addressing the strength of the back. Most often, tightness of the psoas is a reaction to hyperflexion of a spine with weak supporting muscles. Tight hip flexors pull your pelvis far forward, exaggerating the natural lordosis (inward curvature) of your spine.

The Foundation way to counteract psoas tightness is to strengthen the opposing spinal extensor muscles. As these muscles become more powerful, the psoas will move out of spasm and return to an expanded position. A relaxed psoas muscle allows your spine to remain extended while you hinge from the hip. Focusing on extending your spine will get you to a place of strength and reduced pain.

A sedentary lifestyle will shorten your hip flexors, which, of course, affects your lower back. At the same time, contracted hip flexors will stretch your glutes, which then become dormant and cannot properly fire. When this happens, your lower back and hamstrings are forced to compensate. Foundation training is designed to integrate movement using your posterior chain.

THE GLUTEAL MUSCLES

There are three gluteal muscles: gluteus maximus, one of the largest and strongest muscles in the body; gluteus medius; and gluteus minimus. The glutes lift the torso, making us bipedal instead of quadrupedal.

GLUTEUS MAXIMUS

In order for the strong gluteus maximus muscle to contract fully, the lower spine must be in extension, following its natural lordosis. As we have discussed, one obstacle to moving with a flat back or slight flexion is tension in the hip flexors. When the glutes are fully contracted, every standing movement is positively affected, because there is less stress at the hips, knees, and ankles. When the lower spine is extended and the glutes contract, the hip flexors lengthen and relax, the hip joints have minimal compression, and the knee joints are relieved of anterior joint stress, which is the most common cause of degenerative arthritis in the knee.

THE GLUTEUS MEDIUS AND MINIMUS

The gluteus medius is one of two primary abductors of the leg. An abductor pulls the leg sideways, out from the midline of the body. When the feet are planted on the ground, the gluteus medius and gluteus minimus support the pelvis and stabilize the hips.

The gluteus medius is an integral part of back pain diagnoses. When this muscle weakens, the pelvis and hip are unable to sustain balanced standing, walking, or running. Very often, a person with a weak gluteus medius will stand or walk with one foot angled, ducklike.

The gluteus minimus is also known as the hip abductor. This fan-shaped muscle assists in lifting the leg out from the body and rotating the thigh inward. The muscle keeps the pelvis steady when the opposite side is not supported by the leg.

WEAK GLUTES

In general, weak glute muscles create tension in the flexor and internal rotation muscles. Iliacus and psoas muscles are the first line of defense against a weak glute complex. When the glutes protect themselves and contract, the spine and sacrum flex. Building up the strength of the spinal extenders and the glutes will brace the spine and keep it in extension.

THE HAMSTRINGS

Three strong muscles make up the hamstring complex. These muscles attach under the glute muscles and are able to be used with or without the glutes to raise the trunk. Most people are trained to contract the hamstrings from a seated, flexed spine position, which simply does not do justice to the power of these muscles.

Trying to strengthen these important muscles on a leg curling machine at the gym is asking for trouble, as that isolates muscles meant to work with others as a group. Foundation training is about integrated movement. The hamstrings and glutes of the posterior chain should work together for maximal power and minimal risk of injury. When the hip and knee are both slightly flexed, as we teach in all of our Foundation movements, the hamstrings are capable of extending the trunk of the body. When the spine is strong, this movement takes on a whole new meaning.

THE ADDUCTOR GROUP

Three adductor muscles of the inner leg are responsible for moving the thighs toward one another. When the adductor muscles are pulling in too hard, the outer hip muscles are fired up and forced to work too hard. A problem with the iliotibial

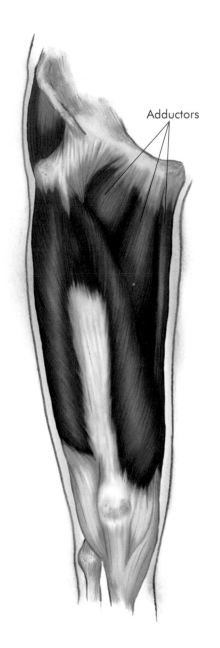

Adductors

Adductor Group

band, or IT band—tendons that attach at the iliac crest, right above the glutes to the bottom of the knee—is a reaction to adductor problems. If the IT band is too tight, you will have outer-knee pain.

When you squeeze your adductor muscles, you can pull your pelvis down and decrease pressure between the discs of your spine. Many Foundation exercises use these muscles as stabilizers.

When the adductor group is too tight, too weak, or chronically in spasm, your back and the inside of your knee hurt. Lengthening and strengthening these muscles will improve movement and reduce back and knee pain. The large muscles of the body are designed for movement. Pain comes from smaller muscles absorbing too much force when the larger ones are used improperly. Foundation training teaches you to use the big muscles for movement.

YOU ARE READY TO MOVE THE RIGHT WAY

With this background, you are ready to get moving the right way. Now that you understand the purpose of these exercises, you will be able to activate the appropriate muscles as you progress through the movements. Don't worry. You don't have to get an advanced degree in anatomy or memorize Latin words to do the workouts. We'll remind you (and show you) what muscles you should be recruiting as we walk you through the workouts. In the next three chapters, we present increasingly demanding Foundation workouts. Be prepared to feel significantly more powerful and to work your way to making back pain a memory.

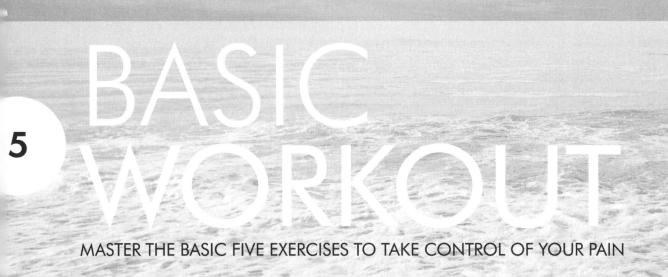

5

BASIC WORKOUT

MASTER THE BASIC FIVE EXERCISES TO TAKE CONTROL OF YOUR PAIN

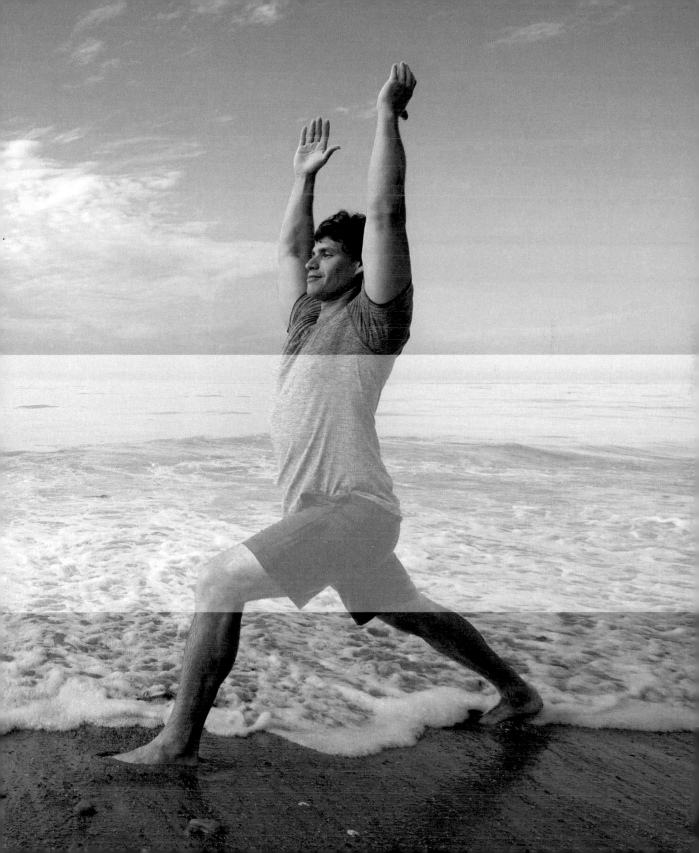

THE BASIC WORKOUT AT A GLANCE

Repeat sequence three times to complete workout.

Time: 15 to 20 minutes

EXERCISE 1: **THE FOUNDER**

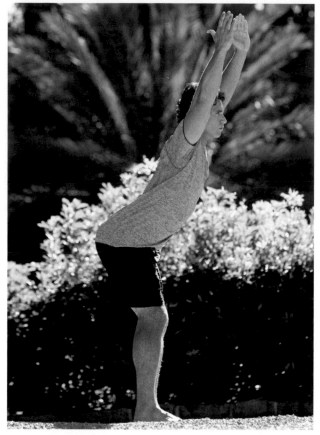

EXERCISE 2: **BACK EXTENSION**

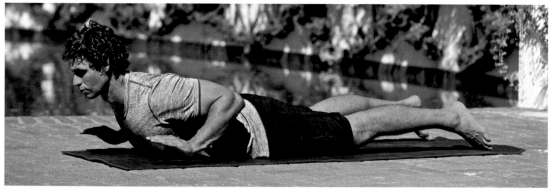

EXERCISE 3: **ADDUCTOR-ASSISTED BACK EXTENSION**

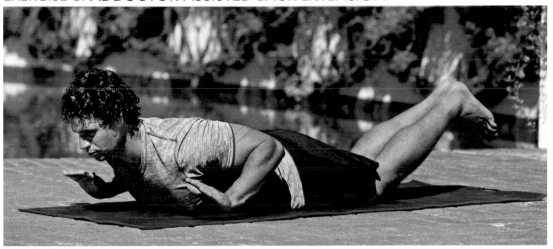

EXERCISE 4: **CHILD'S POSE/ KNEELING FOUNDER**

EXERCISE 5: **LUNGE STRETCH**

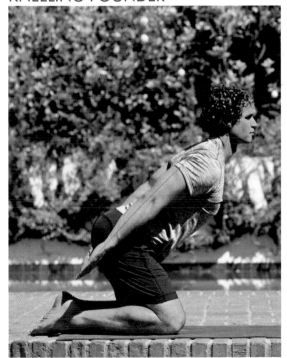

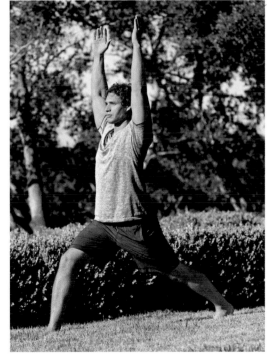

People suffering with acute back pain usually just want to lie down and rest. When you are in extreme pain, movement can be scary. You do not want to risk hurting yourself more. An acute injury may require a day or two of rest, and the hardest part of feeling better is taking the first step. Movement is challenging if you really hurt, but there's little else that will put you on the road to wellness more quickly than moving correctly. Often, with the intention of preventing further back injury, doctors

The only way to get the muscles to relax is to move, functionally transferring the stress that is causing the injury or inflammation in your back to your posterior chain, which is built to take it, and thereby relieving the pain.

will prescribe prolonged bed rest and limit all activities. We would not say that this is the wrong approach, but it certainly does not accelerate the healing process. Though it may seem counterintuitive, proper movement—even when you are in pain—is the most effective remedy. Extended bed rest will only make your muscles weaker, and, as you have learned, pain is the price you pay for weak muscles.

Muscle spasms cause pain, but they function as a warning sign: Something else is going wrong with your body mechanics. Back spasms are defense mechanisms; the muscles contract, protecting a deeper problem. The only way to get the muscles to relax is to move, functionally transferring the stress that is causing the injury or inflammation in your back to your posterior chain, which is built to take it, and thereby relieving the pain.

WHEN TO SEE A MEDICAL PROFESSIONAL

If you are having back pain for the first time and have no idea what is wrong with your back, have it checked by a doctor of chiropractic or an osteopathic or medical doctor before doing Foundation training or any new regimen.

The Foundation program at the heart of this book consists of three 2-week workouts that correspond to different levels of back pain and rehabilitation, as well as difficulty: a basic workout for acute pain, a moderate workout for chronic pain, and a more intense workout for prevention and strengthening during pain-free periods. We also include two bonus exercises for added flexibility, targeting tightness and pain in the hips, pelvis, and upper legs.

The goal of the three workouts is to build layer upon layer of stronger back muscles to brace your spine and lengthen the muscles in the front of your body. These exercises are designed to recruit the posterior chain muscles to work together. Foundation training is about integrated movement.

The exercises you are about to try are body-weight resistance exercises specifically designed to challenge and strengthen your back. Foundation training, unlike conventional resistance training, is based on holding challenging postures that promote a unique combination of strength and flexibility. Move through the indi-

FOUNDATIONFIRST

Rob Lowe, actor

Let me tell you that these guys have created something serious. Until you do the work, it is hard to understand how strong you can become through body-weight training. Not only am I in the best shape of my life, but my body moves and feels completely different. I feel stronger in everything I do.

vidual exercises in a smoothly flowing progression, and then repeat the series as directed.

The exercises are simple, but you won't be accustomed to the movements and will probably feel awkward at first. Since you'll be activating muscles you usually do not work so hard, your body will probably start to shake. Don't worry about it. Even the strongest professional athletes shake when they train with us, and they begin with the basics just like you.

Though the exercises are easy to learn and you can breeze through them, they are hard. Done correctly, these movements strain you and stress your body. You can blow through them, of course, but you will not be getting the full benefits of the workout. The difference between hard and easy is the amount of time the muscles are under tension and how much you push it. Find the spot that is tightest on your body, go deep, and work through it. To work through pain, you have to be strong. To progress, you have to work harder. Be aware of your breath. Breathing deeply will help you hold the stretch.

We created the first workout to fix your pain. The first 2 weeks focus purely on training your back and hips to hinge properly while opening and relaxing the hip flexor muscles. The five basic exercises provide a foundation for movement and power in the future. These exercises represent the fundamental Foundation training movements. The more time you take to develop that first level of strength and

endurance, the longer the benefits will last. We recommend that you do the exercises for the basic workout for 15 to 20 minutes at least three days a week.

The first 2 weeks focus purely on training your back and hips to hinge properly while opening and relaxing the hip flexor muscles. The five basic exercises provide a foundation for movement and power in the future.

Form is very important if you want results, so learn to do the exercises the right way. We troubleshoot each movement by illustrating and explaining common mistakes that will make the exercise less effective. We also use photo illustrations to identify the muscle groups being worked for each exercise in the workout, so you will know where you should be feeling the tension.

If you take the time to learn to do the basic five properly, you will be set for the rest of your life. Just as you can hop on a bike and pedal away even if you have not ridden in years, your body will remember the positions. You will be able to do this workout quickly and easily, without having to refer to anything. Anytime your back goes out, you will not have to run to the doctor or be out of commission. You can do these basic exercises to break through your pain and get back on track.

Give us 2 weeks and you will feel a substantial difference in how you move and a reduction in back pain. We would not say this if we had not seen these results with all of our clients. They cannot believe how quickly the benefits appear. They report that they feel as if they have a brace tightening up the muscles around the spine. Their hamstrings are stronger and more flexible. In almost every case, they immediately begin to feel good again.

> Give us 2 weeks and you will feel a substantial difference in how you move and a reduction in back pain.

The basic exercises were designed to eliminate pain quickly. Once you cross the pain bridge, you progress to building strength and reinforcing the movements. If you do not feel a change after 2 weeks of doing the basic five, either you are doing the exercises incorrectly or you should see a doctor.

Most rehabilitation focuses on one muscle and one movement, but the five basic Foundation exercises work on gross movement rather than one or two joints. These exercises work to activate all your muscles together.

As you do the basic sequence, you should flow from one movement to the next, one exercise to the other. Your muscles have memory; training will help solidify and reinforce this memory, and the movements you do in these exercises will carry over into every move you make all day long. When your movement patterns change, you stop aggravating your back problems. To complete the workout, repeat these exercises in sequence three times.

THE BASIC WORKOUT
EXERCISE 1
THE FOUNDER

This exercise works the entire posterior chain. You are activating your glutes, hamstrings, lower back, and upper back.

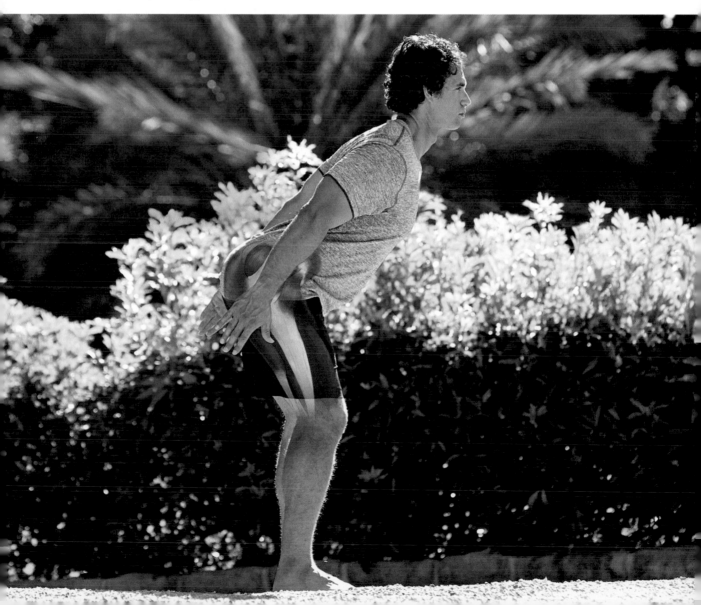

THE FOUNDER

The Founder is the basis for all Foundation movement. We designed the exercise to teach you correct movement patterns. The Founder strengthens the deepest muscles in your spine, which hold your spine in extension. The exercise actually consists of several movements that flow from one to another.

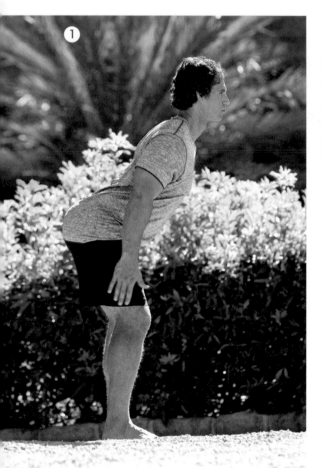
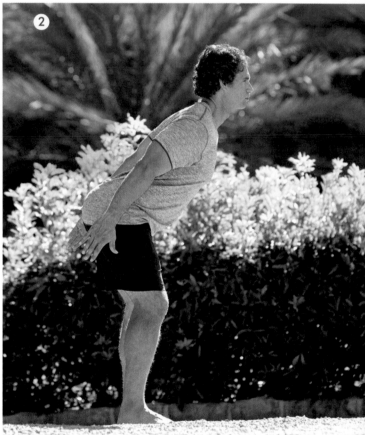

1 Stand with your feet shoulder-width apart. Bend your knees slightly. Keep your weight on your heels. Extend your spine by hinging from your hips.

2 Reach back with your arms, shoulders pulling down toward your butt. Really think of pushing your hips back and feeling the tension in your lower back. Hold this position for 15 seconds.

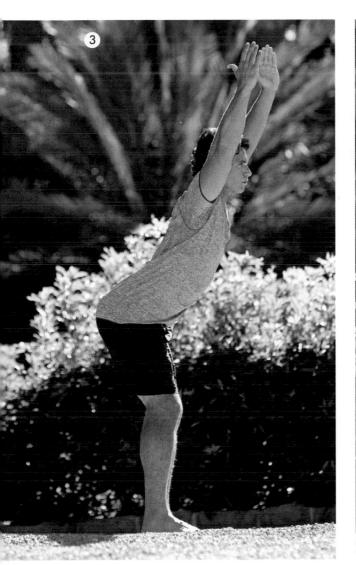 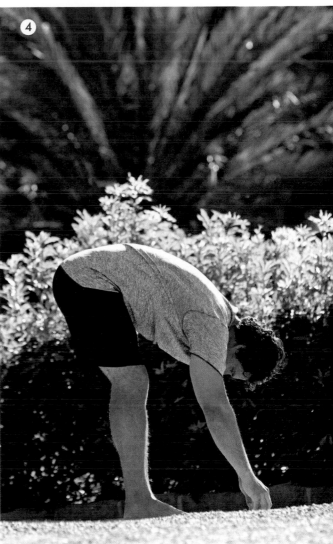

3 Stay in this position and lift your arms in front of you as high as you can. Keep your weight on your heels and your hips back. Hold this position for 15 seconds.

4 Take a deep breath. As you exhale, fold all the way forward, keeping your back flat. Make sure your knees are slightly bent and your weight remains on your heels. Take two deep breaths while stretching.

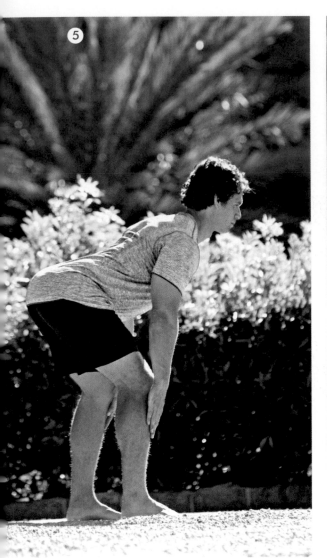 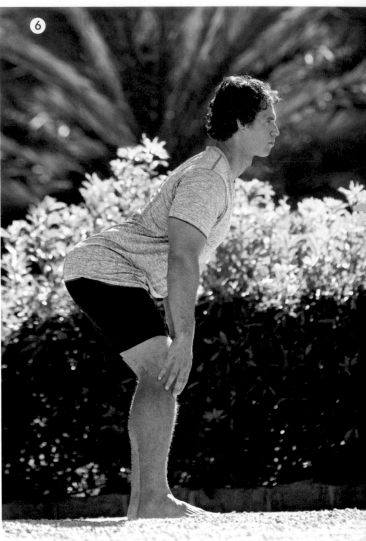

⑤ Very important: Bend your knees another couple of inches. Press your hands against your shins. Look up. Extend your spine, chest high. Pull your shoulders back and arch your lower back. Hold this position for 15 seconds.

⑥ Keeping your back extended, slide your hands up to your knees.

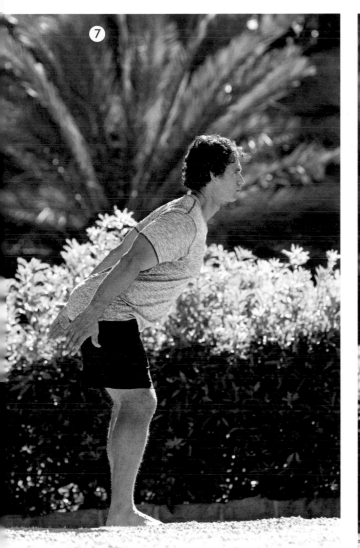
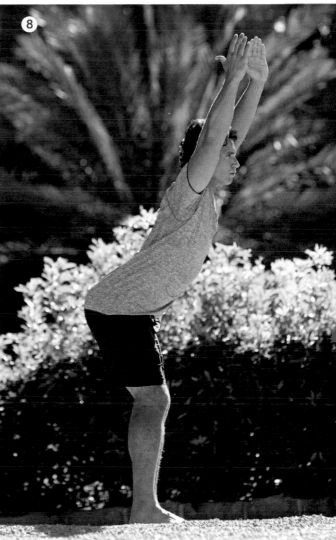

7 Push your arms behind you and squeeze your shoulder blades together, assuming the starting position. Keep your spine extended and your weight on your heels. Hold for 15 seconds.

8 Lift your arms in front of you as high as you can. Hold this position for 20 seconds or four deep breaths.

THE PERFECT FOUNDER

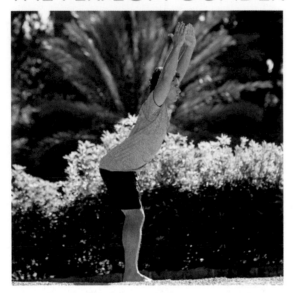

- Keep your head up, looking straight ahead.
- Extend your lower spine by lifting your chest and pushing your butt backward.
- Keep your weight on your heels.
- Stick your butt back as far as possible without falling over.
- When you lift your arms, keep them close to your ears.

TROUBLESHOOTING THE FOUNDER

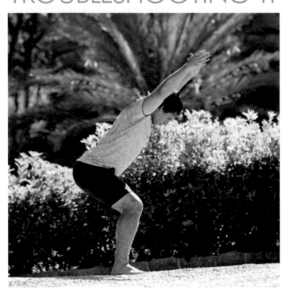

- Head looks down rather than straight ahead.
- Knees are too far forward. They should be over the ankles, not the toes.
- Weight is on the balls of feet instead of heels.
- Arms are spread too wide.

EXERCISE 2
BACK EXTENSION (15 REPS)

This exercise reinforces a good back extension by working the muscles that brace your spine, the erector spinae and multifidi. By pulling your elbows as far back as you can, toward your butt, you will tighten your midback, and the position will pull you into a forceful extension. This is a real strengthener that stabilizes muscles at the base of the spine.

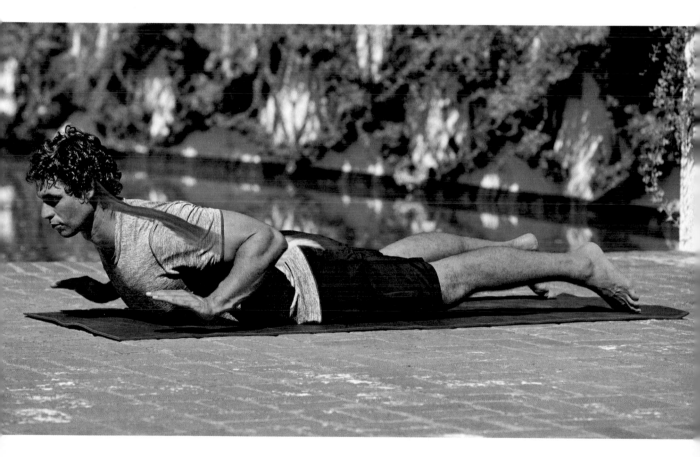

BACK EXTENSION

The repetitive contraction and relaxation of this back extension with a shoulder blade squeeze will begin to block pain receptors. This exercise is a strengthener that stabilizes the muscles at the base of your spine. When the back is acting up, we've found this exercise is the most effective of the group.

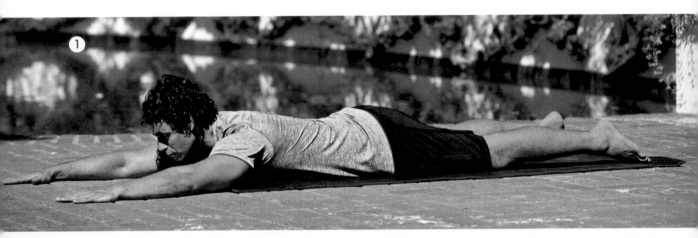

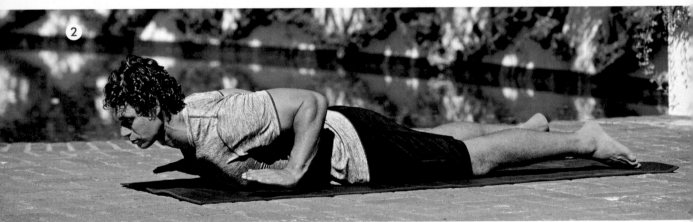

① Lie flat on your stomach with your arms stretched out in front of you. Look at the floor a few inches in front of you; do not extend your neck to look straight ahead.

② Bring your elbows and forearms off the floor, and pull your elbows hard into your rib cage/ midback, using your shoulder blades. You will contract your shoulder blades hard throughout the entire exercise, causing your chest to rise and your neck to lengthen.

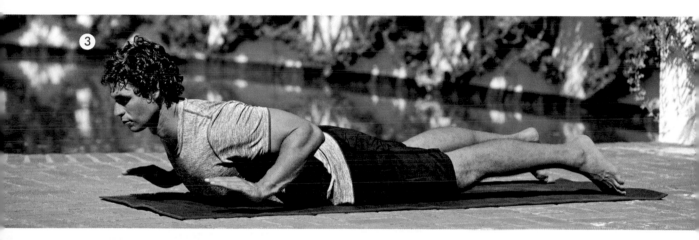

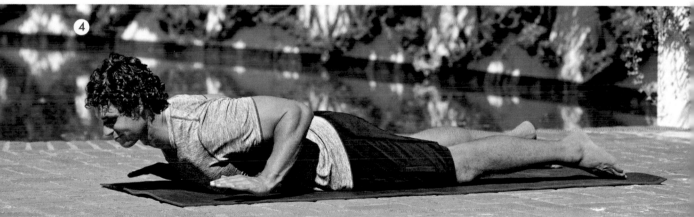

3 Lift your upper body off the floor, leading with your chest. Keep your feet flat on the ground to avoid excess spinal compression.

4 Slowly lower your chest while keeping your elbows and hands off the ground.

Repeat 15 times.

THE PERFECT BACK EXTENSION

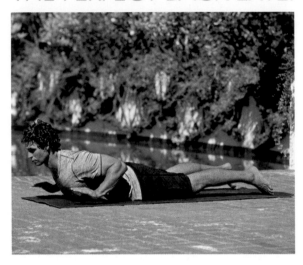

- Feet stay on the ground.
- Arms and elbows are pulled tight against the body.
- Elbows are pulled back toward the butt.
- Spine is in alignment.
- Shoulders are down.

TROUBLESHOOTING THE BACK EXTENSION

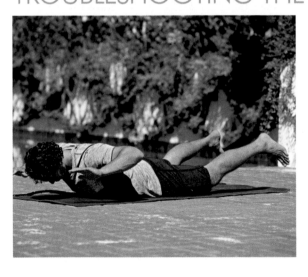

- Arms are too far forward and elbows are not close to the body, which will raise the shoulders and significantly increase the stress on the lower spine.
- Legs rise as the back is pulled up.

EXERCISE 3
ADDUCTOR-ASSISTED BACK
EXTENSION (10- TO 20-SECOND HOLDS)

This exercise works a number of important muscle groups: adductors, erector spinae, hamstrings, and glutes. The movement is unique in that by contracting the adductor muscles, you are actually tractioning the pelvis and, ultimately, the lower spine. This helps alleviate the compression of many lower-back issues.

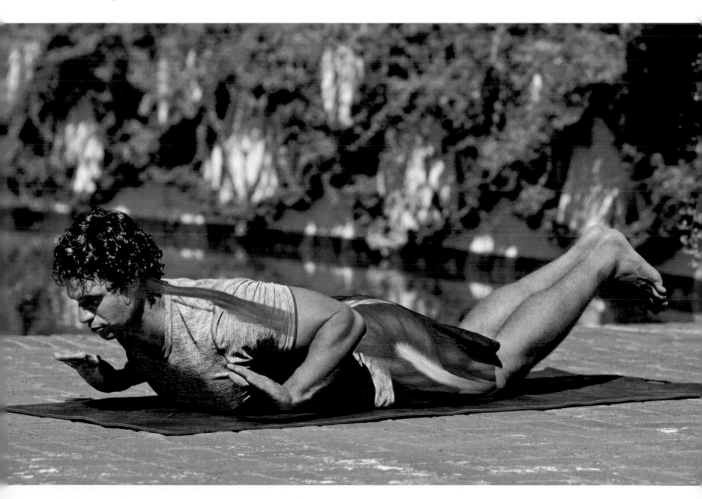

ADDUCTOR-ASSISTED BACK EXTENSION

This back extension with raised and squeezed legs works the adductor muscles inside your thighs. The adductors originate in the pelvis and attach to the knee. Contracting these muscles pulls the pelvis down and alleviates compression of the lower spine.

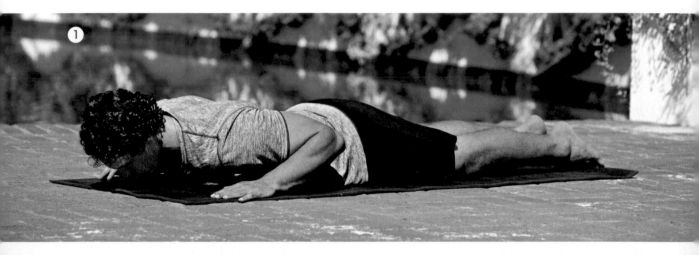

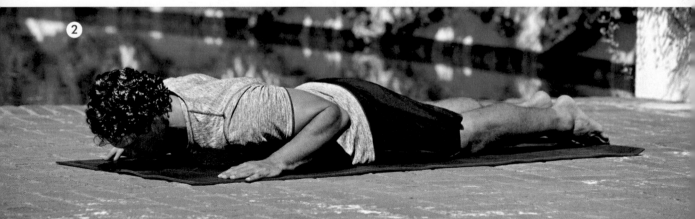

1 Lie flat on your stomach with your palms on the floor by your shoulders.

2 Pull your elbows back against your rib cage and your arms up off the ground. Bring your feet and knees together firmly.

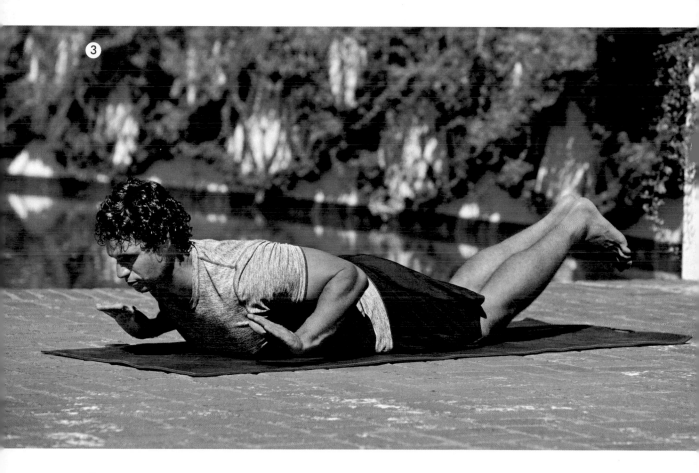

3 Bend your knees to a 45-degree angle while pressing your knees and feet together as tightly as possible. Lower your feet until they are 6 inches off the ground. Lift your chest as high as you can while you continue to hold your feet 6 inches off the ground. Hold the pose for 10 to 20 seconds. The more you squeeze your knees together, the better this exercise is for you.

THE PERFECT ADDUCTOR-ASSISTED BACK EXTENSION

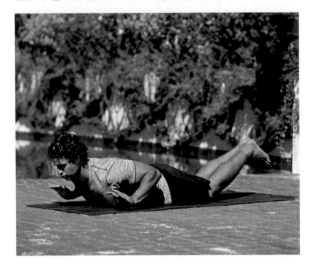

- This exercise is most effective when the knees are pressed firmly together. Most people simply bend their knees and lift both legs off the ground.

- Your legs should be bent so your feet are only 6 inches off the ground.

- Do not hyperextend the neck. Look at the floor a few inches in front of you.

TROUBLESHOOTING THE ADDUCTOR-ASSISTED BACK EXTENSION

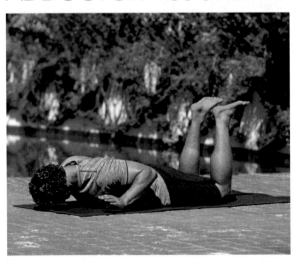

- Arms are too far forward and elbows are not close to the body, which raises the shoulders toward the ears and significantly increases the stress on the lower spine.

- Knees and feet are not pressed together, which diminishes the effect of the exercise.

EXERCISE 4
CHILD'S POSE/
KNEELING FOUNDER

This exercise uses the erector spinae, glutes, and quadratus lumborum. The exercise is designed to teach your body to go from flexion to extension.

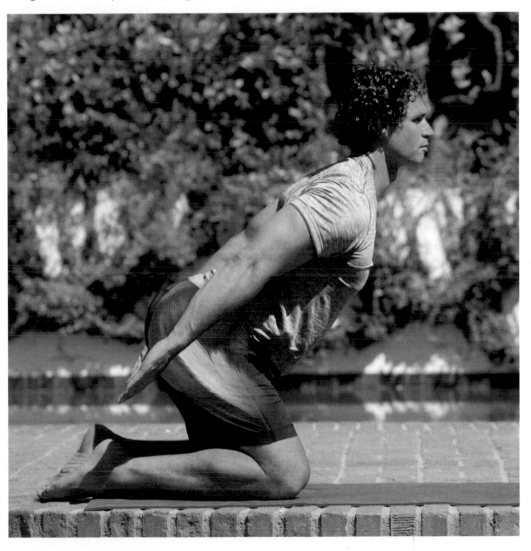

CHILD'S POSE/KNEELING FOUNDER

This exercise will teach your body to go from flexion to extension. First you put your back into a flexion stretch, then you engage in an active contraction of the posterior chain muscles. When you raise your arms, you will isolate tension at your lower spine. You will be able to flex farther at the hip joints and isolate your lower-back muscles. If you feel any pain in your knees, refrain from doing this exercise.

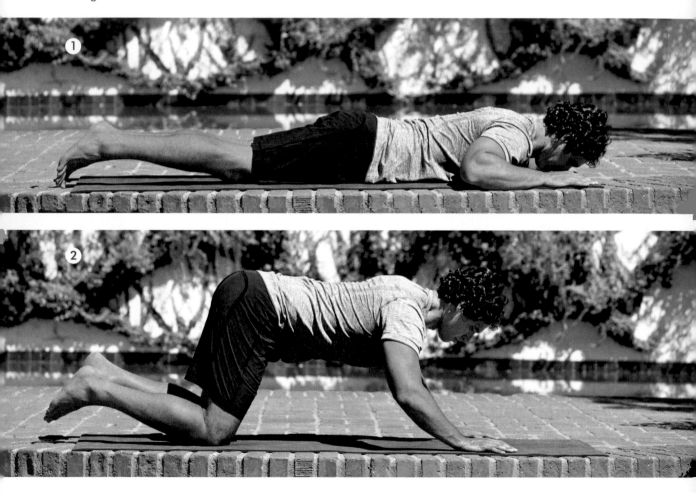

1 Begin on your stomach with your palms on the floor by your ears.

2 Bend your knees and pull your hips all the way back to your heels.

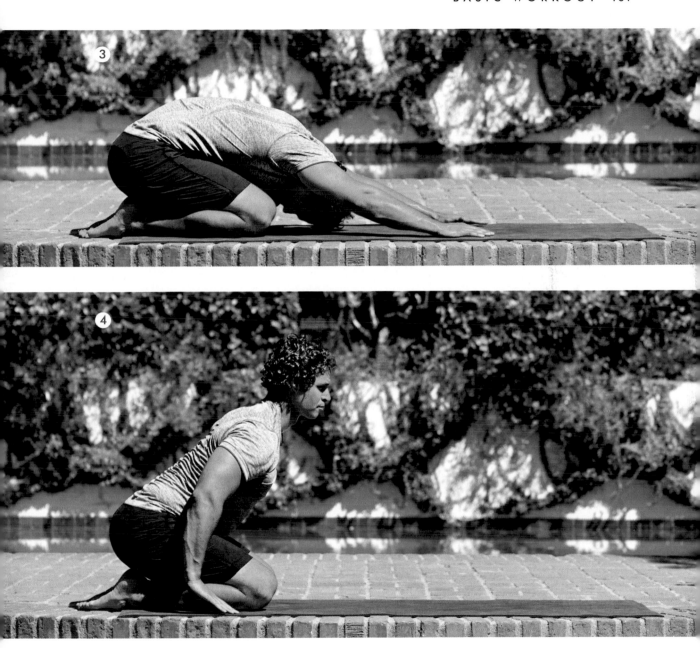

③ Hold this position for 20 to 30 seconds.

④ Begin to lift your chest with your butt still resting on your heels.

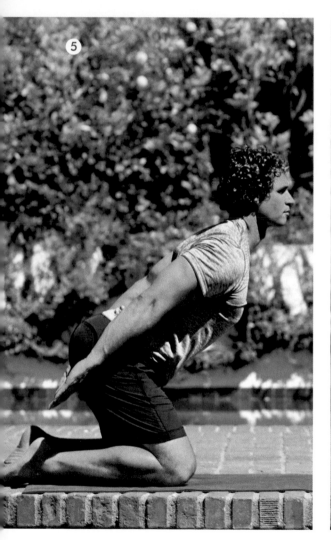

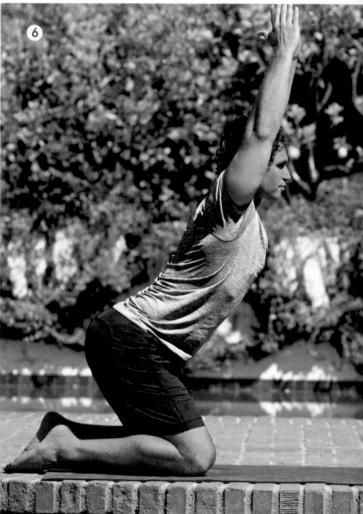

5 Lift your butt off your heels, keeping your chest high and back extended. Reach back with your arms, shoulders pulling down toward your butt. Press your chest forward as far as you can. Hold for 10 to 15 seconds.

6 Slowly lift your arms all the way up in front of you while supporting yourself with your back and hips. Hold this position for 10 seconds.

THE PERFECT CHILD'S POSE/ KNEELING FOUNDER

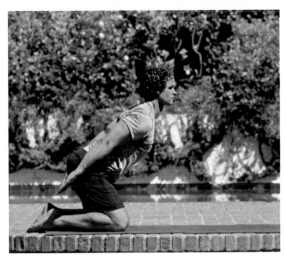

- Head is up, looking straight ahead.
- Lower spine is extended by lifting chest and pushing butt backward.
- Hips stay back just above heels; hips do not press forward.
- Lifted arms are held close to ears.

TROUBLESHOOTING THE CHILD'S POSE/ KNEELING FOUNDER

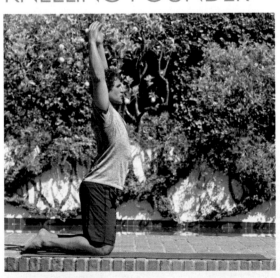

- The back is flexed and not strongly extended.
- Hips come too far forward.
- Torso is straight instead of leaning forward.

EXERCISE 5
LUNGE STRETCH
(HOLD 20 SECONDS PER SIDE)

This exercise stretches the opposing muscles, the ilipsoas and quadratus lumborum muscles. It is a very powerful active stretch for the antagonist muscles generally associated with back pain. The hips make the whole body more flexible. These muscles are not isolated: They are connected to the back. When you stretch these muscles, your glutes are not jammed into your hip, and they do not have to pull hard. We like to end a workout with a Lunge Stretch, because it opens you up and allows your back to remain in its natural curved position throughout the day.

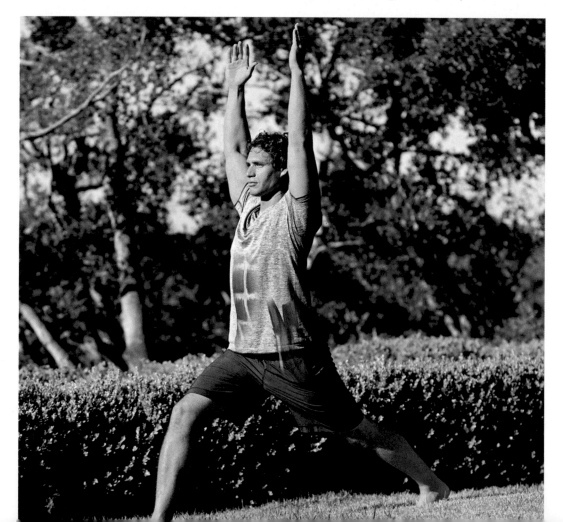

LUNGE STRETCH

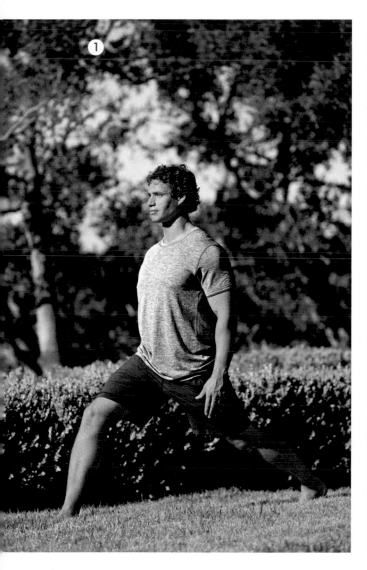

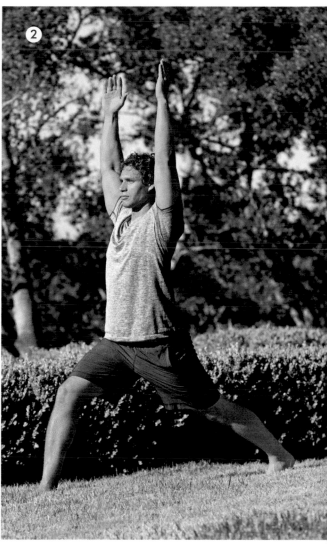

1 Get into a long lunge with your right leg forward, knee slightly bent. Make sure your right knee is pressed behind your ankle, not over your toes. Keep your left foot facing forward and your back heel pressing toward the ground.

2 Extend your spine from the hips and raise your arms overhead. As you extend, you should feel a stretch at the hip flexors of the back leg.

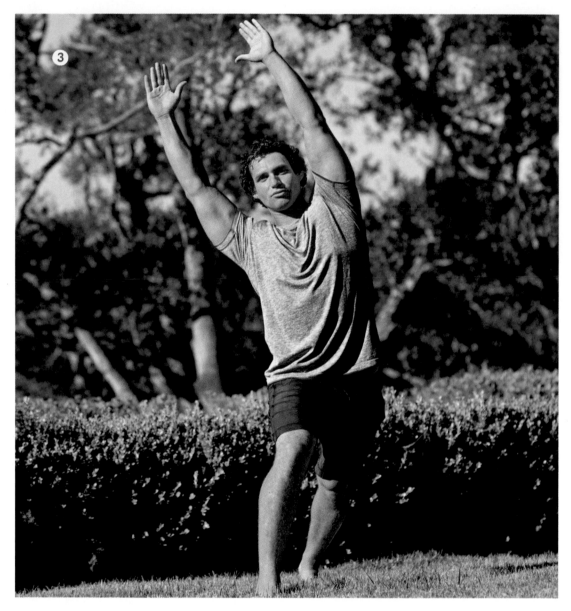

3 Laterally flex your upper body to the right, away from your left (or back) leg, while keeping extension in your spine. Keep your hips squared. Hold the stretch for 20 seconds.

Repeat the stretch with your left leg bent forward and your right leg extended behind you. Flex your upper body to the left and hold for 20 seconds.

THE PERFECT LUNGE STRETCH

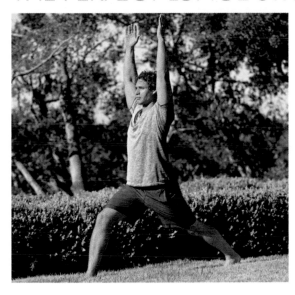

- Back is extended.
- Arms are straight up.
- Shoulders are down.
- Front knee is pressed back behind the ankle.
- Hips remain squared, even with the bend.

TROUBLESHOOTING THE LUNGE STRETCH

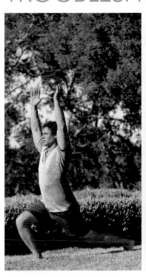 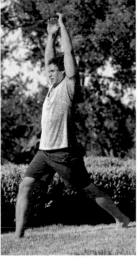

- All of the weight is shifted forward on the ball of the front foot.
- Shoulders are raised toward ears.
- The lunging knee is too far forward over the foot.
- Hips are not squared.

When you have completed the fifth exercise, go back to the Founder and cycle through this basic workout two more times.

That is the first 2 weeks of the program. We know it's repetitive, but repetition is required to master the movements and move forward . . . literally. You have learned the basics of Foundation training, which will help free you from acute pain.

The exercises may not have seemed challenging when you first flipped through these pages, but if you did them correctly, you soon learned how challenging they are. You have been targeting the exact muscles you need to brace your spine, and you felt your posterior chain activating. When you can feel it in your body, you get it. We've seen many people experience this aha moment once they've activated the correct muscles.

Try to make the routine part of your lifestyle. Many of our clients do these exercises every day when they get out of bed in the morning. It increases their awareness of their bodies and hits the on switch for the right muscles, programming them to move well throughout the day. This quick workout reinforces the movement patterns that will allow people to live pain free.

In the course of 2 weeks, you should notice that your pain has eased up, your back feels stronger, and your posture is changing. A flexed spine and inner rotation begin to feel slightly uncomfortable. If you are not feeling an improvement after 2 weeks, you should evaluate what you are doing. Your form might not be right. Be sure to refer to the troubleshooting directions for each exercise. If that checks out, you should consult with your doctor. You may have an underlying problem that requires medical attention.

As your acute pain becomes less intense, support your Foundation work with easy exercise. Walk, get on a bike, just keep moving. Staying active will keep your muscles healthy. Now that your movement patterns are changing, your posterior chain and hips will do the work and remove the stress and friction on your spine that have been responsible for your pain. You have corrected the source of your problems and strengthened your back at the same time. This double achievement will prevent future relapses. You should now be sufficiently out of pain so that you can turn up the intensity and move on to the moderate workout in the next chapter.

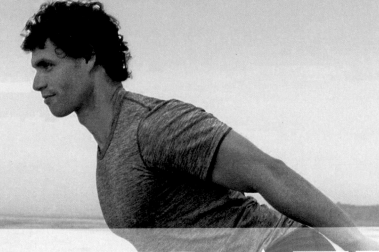

6 MODERATE WORKOUT

BUILDING ON THE BASICS

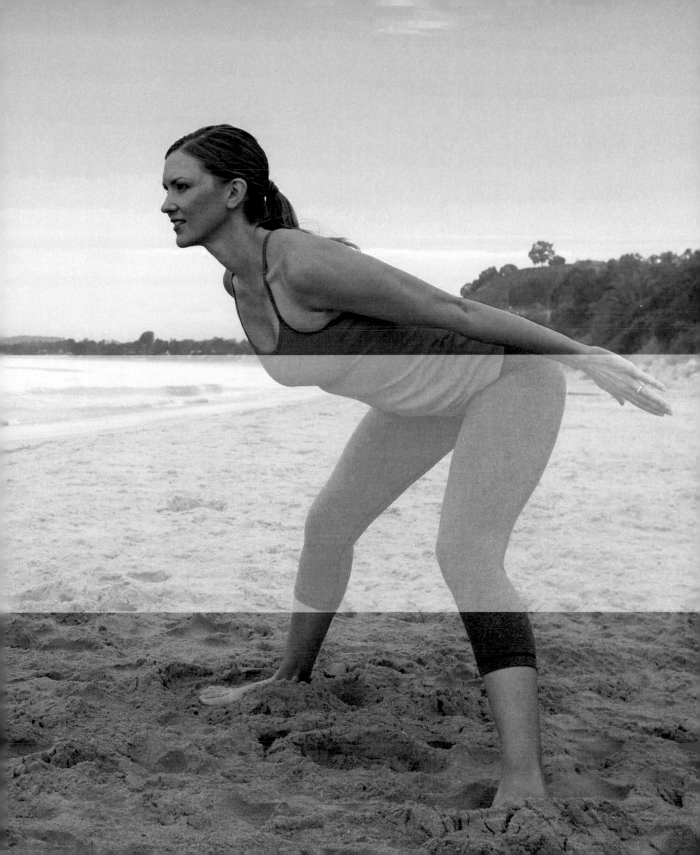

THE MODERATE WORKOUT AT A GLANCE

Repeat sequence three times to complete workout.

Time: 30 minutes

EXERCISE 1: THE FOUNDER

EXERCISE 2: FOUNDATION SQUAT

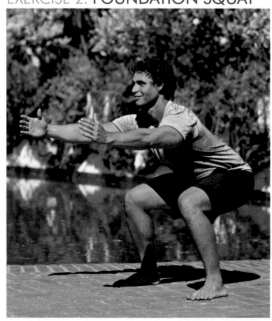

EXERCISE 3: WOODPECKER

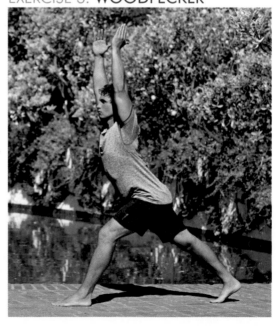

EXERCISE 4: BACK EXTENSION

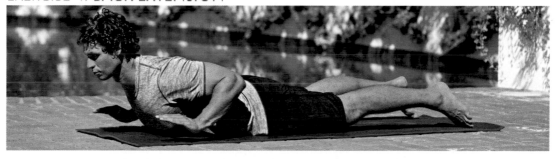

EXERCISE 5: ADDUCTOR-ASSISTED BACK EXTENSION

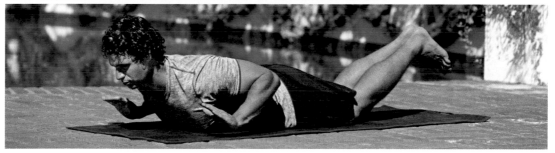

EXERCISE 6: CHILD'S POSE/ KNEELING FOUNDER

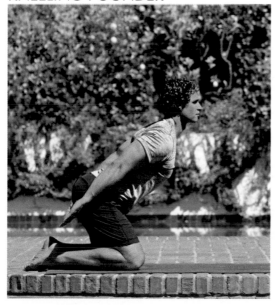

EXERCISE 7: LUNGE STRETCH

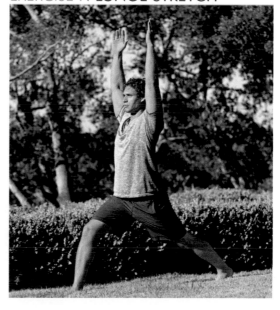

The moderate workout is designed to help you deal with pain that lasts or keeps coming back. These exercises will transform your nagging, restricting back pain to vigorous freedom of movement. It might be unrealistic to expect to be totally pain free all the time, but as you become stronger, your proportionate response will be faster. If your back pain should return, you will be able to get it under control quickly.

You'll turn up the intensity and further your progress by adding two exercises to the basic workout. This workout will tone your muscles and increase your flexibility by adding more torque and angles to the movements.

When you have done this level of Foundation training for 2 weeks, you will become more conscious of your back muscles and how you are using them. Many of our clients tell us that for the first time, they are aware of how the muscles of their lower spine work.

Repeat this sequence of seven exercises three times. It should take you around 30 minutes to complete. Concentrate on where you feel the tightness in your body as you do the exercises. Now that you have learned the movements, try to get deeper into each position when you do the five exercises from the basic workout. Push your hips back farther, lift your arms higher, and contract your lower-back muscles harder. Once you feel the stretch while you are in an extended position, take a deep breath and bend more from the hips. Challenging yourself will pay off.

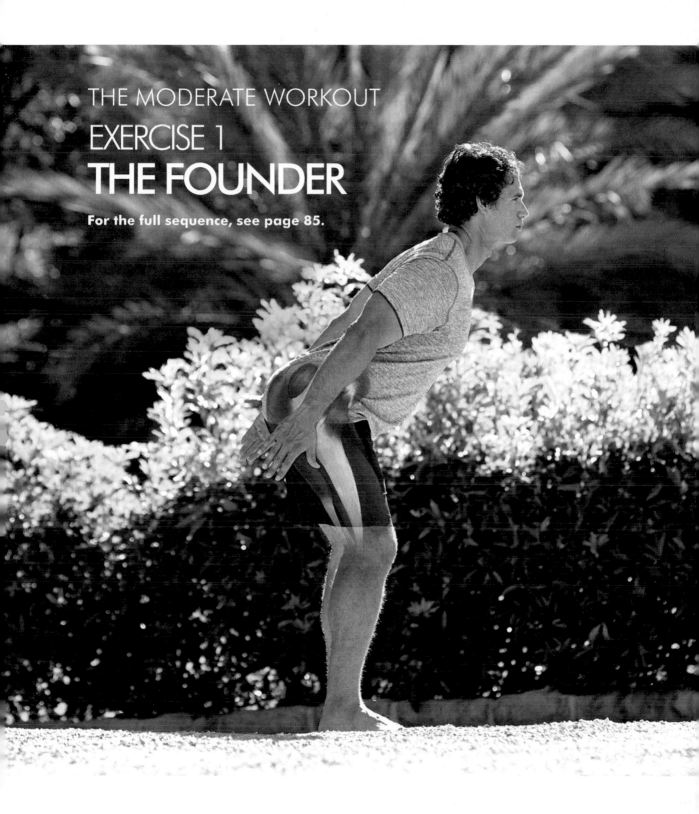

THE MODERATE WORKOUT
EXERCISE 1
THE FOUNDER

For the full sequence, see page 85.

EXERCISE 2
FOUNDATION SQUAT (10 REPS)

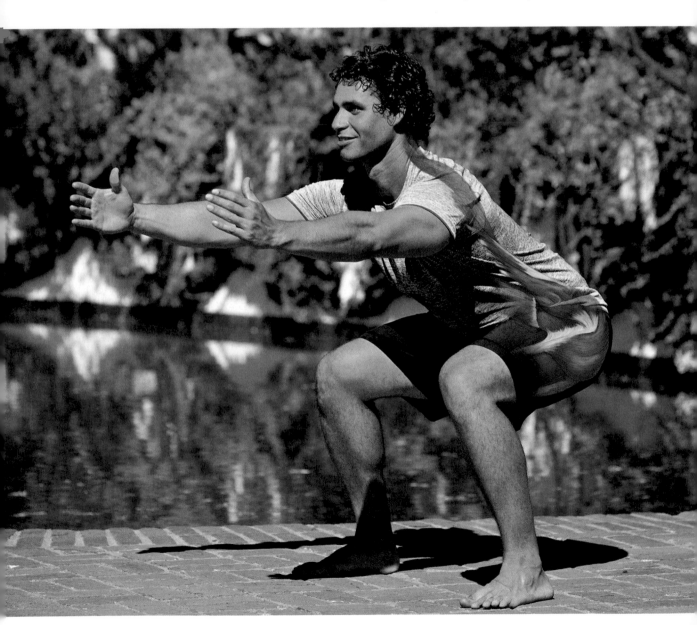

FOUNDATION SQUAT

The Foundation Squat is a surprisingly easy exercise to learn and will yield remarkable results. It is all about the hinge. In fact, this is an essential exercise for developing the hinge. The movement primarily works the glutes and erector spinae.

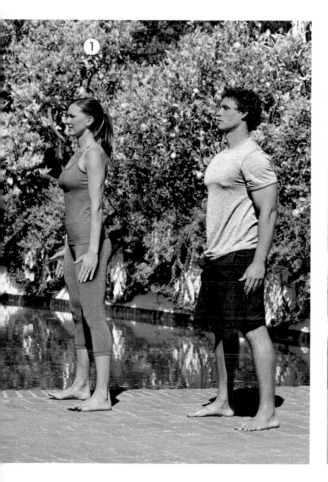 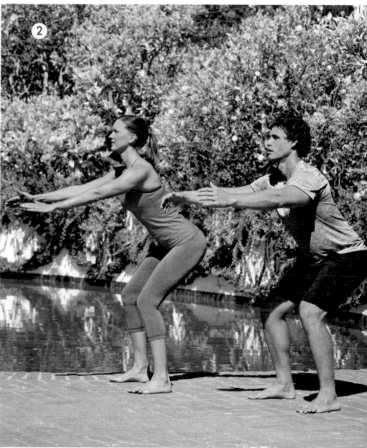

1 Stand with your feet slightly more than shoulder-width apart. Keep your weight far back on your heels. Work on pushing your heels into the ground, as if you are trying to spread the floor apart.

2 Bring your arms out in front as you begin pushing your butt behind you. Keep your back in extension.

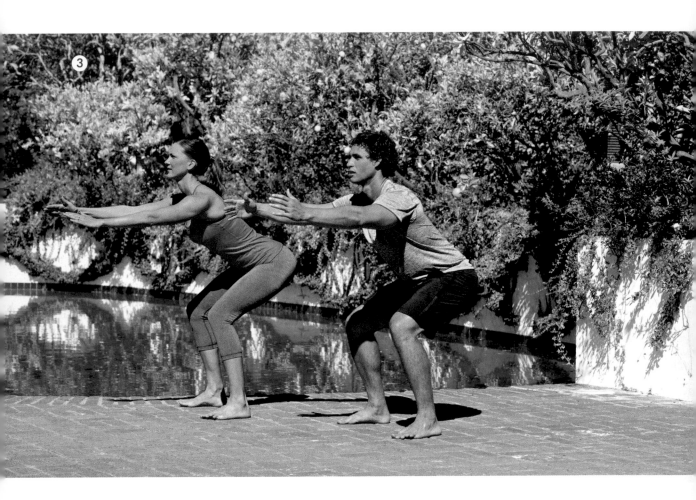

3 Keep pressing your butt back as you continue to bend your knees deeper into the squat. As you pull into the squat, use your hip flexors.

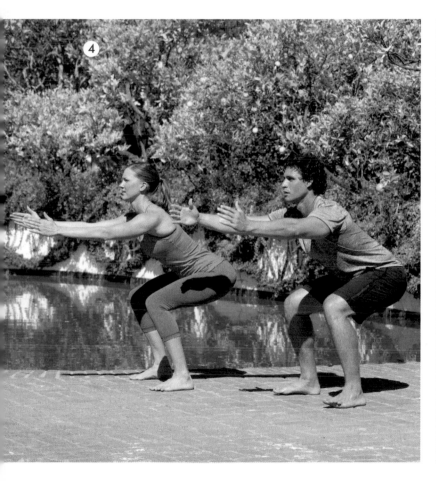
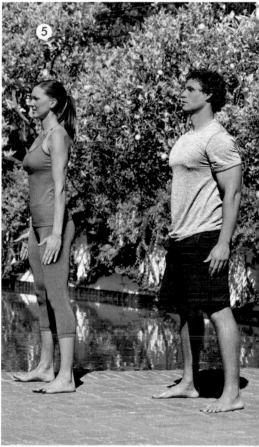

4 Continue to lower yourself until your knees are bent about 90 degrees. Your knees should never come past the front of your feet.

5 Pressing up through your heels, come back up to the starting position with your arms by your sides. Repeat this in a smooth flowing motion 10 times in all.

THE PERFECT FOUNDATION SQUAT

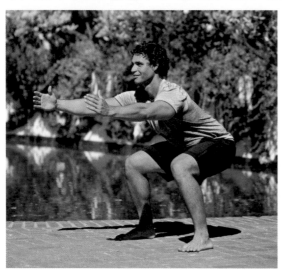

- Back is going to be a bit flexed.
- Chest is high.
- Butt is pushed way back.
- Weight is on the heels.

TROUBLESHOOTING THE FOUNDATION SQUAT

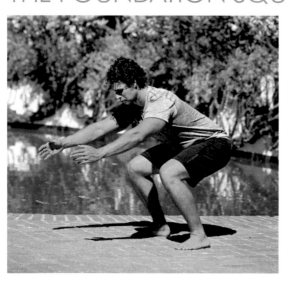

- Weight is forward on toes.
- Back is rounded.
- Spine is too flexed.
- Knees are too far forward.

EXERCISE 3
WOODPECKER

The Woodpecker works your glutes, hamstrings, and erector spinae. By focusing movement in the upper hamstrings, this exercise is very effective in removing pressure from your knees.

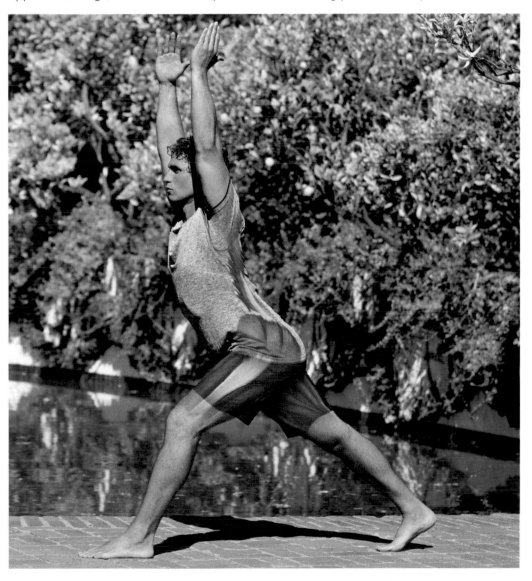

WOODPECKER

The Woodpecker is designed to introduce movement from the upper hamstrings, and it will prepare you to learn a new movement pattern. This exercise alleviates pressure from the knees and is one of the miracle moves when done the right way.

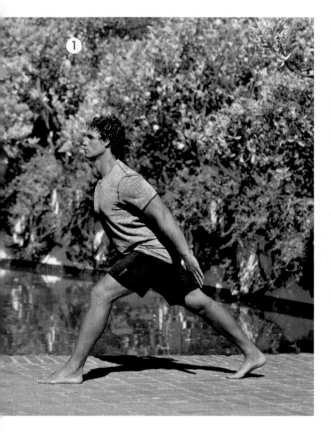
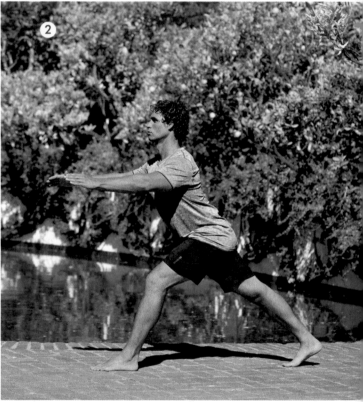

1 Step forward into a lunge with your front knee slightly bent and hips squared. Place your arms by your sides.

2 Keeping your back braced and your shoulders pulled back, begin to hinge forward from the hips, moving your arms straight in front of you. Pretend there is a string attached to your sternum and your upper body is being pulled forward, not down. You will feel a stretch at the upper hamstring and glute of the front leg.

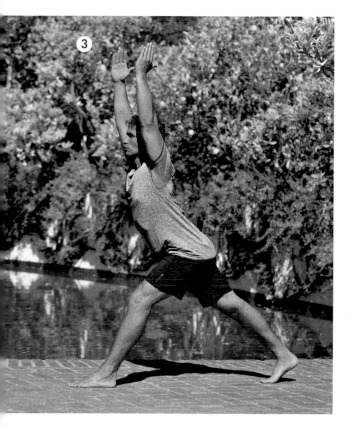
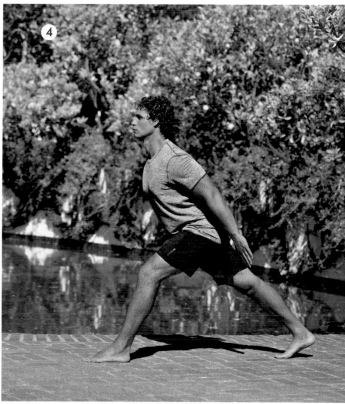

③ Once you feel a good stretch, try to contract your glutes and upper hamstring by pressing your front heel into the ground. Slowly lift your arms in front of you as high as you can, and hold this position for 20 seconds.

④ Then extend your spine further and press your arms behind you, just like in the Founder.

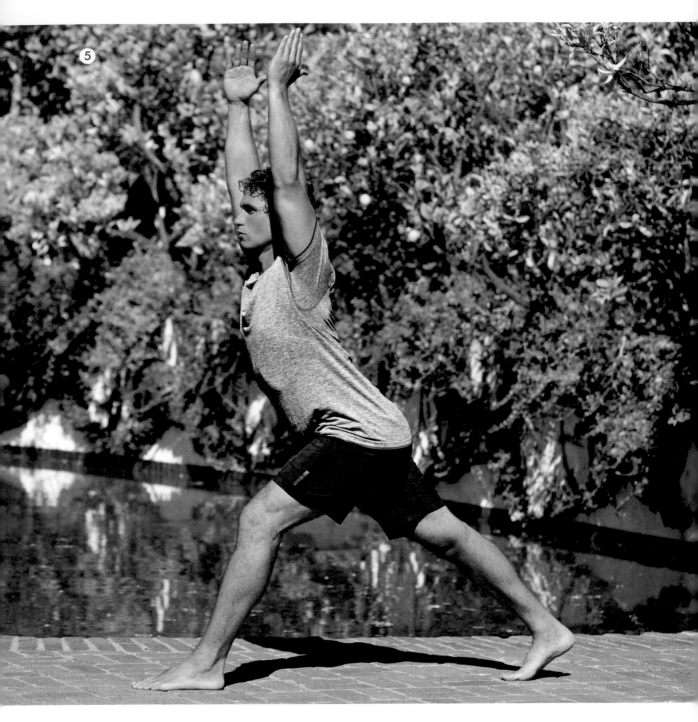

5 Keeping the rest of your body in the same position, slowly raise your arms all the way up in front of you. Hold for 15 seconds.

THE PERFECT WOODPECKER

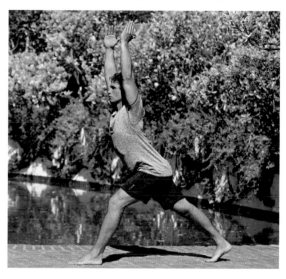

- Hold chest up, shoulders back.
- Hinge from the hips.
- Keep hips squared.
- Keep front knee over ankle.

TROUBLESHOOTING THE WOODPECKER

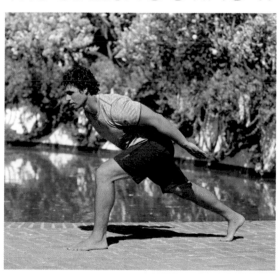

- Back is rounded.
- Hinge from lower back.
- Hips are angled.
- Front knee is too far forward.

EXERCISE 4
BACK EXTENSION (15 REPS)

Try to make your movements stronger to increase the range of extension, but remember to keep your feet on the floor.

(For the full sequence, see page 91.)

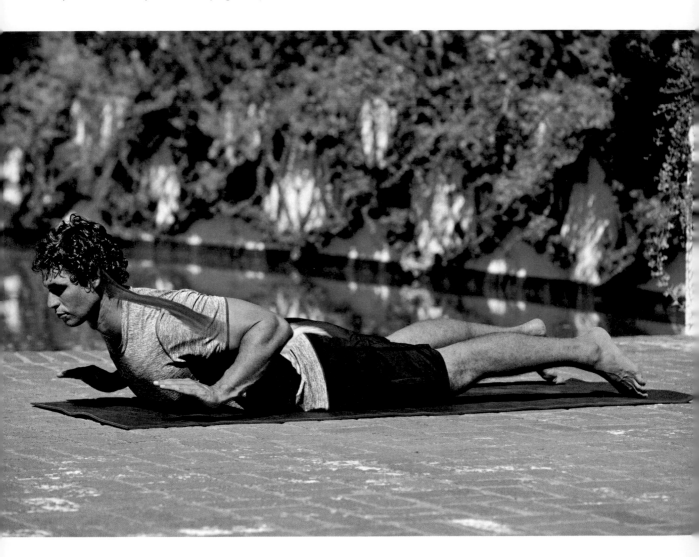

EXERCISE 5
ADDUCTOR-ASSISTED BACK EXTENSION
(20- TO 30-SECOND HOLDS)

(For the full sequence, see page 95.)

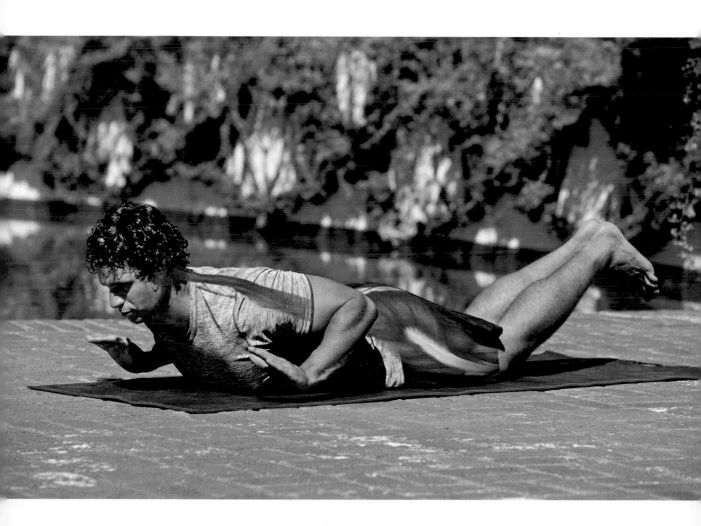

EXERCISE 6
CHILD'S POSE/
KNEELING FOUNDER

(For the full sequence, see page 99.)

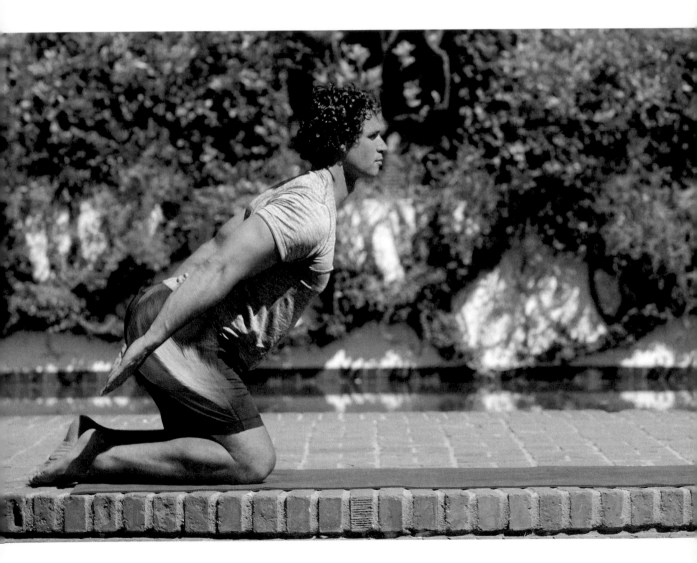

EXERCISE 7
LUNGE STRETCH
(HOLD 20 SECONDS PER SIDE)

(For the full sequence, see page 104.)

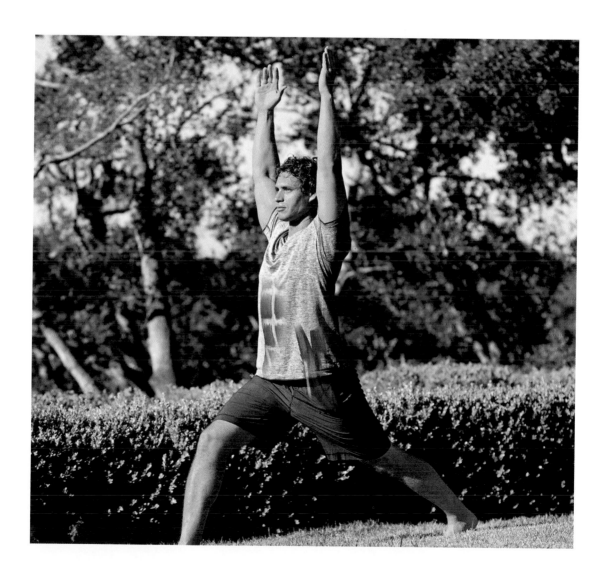

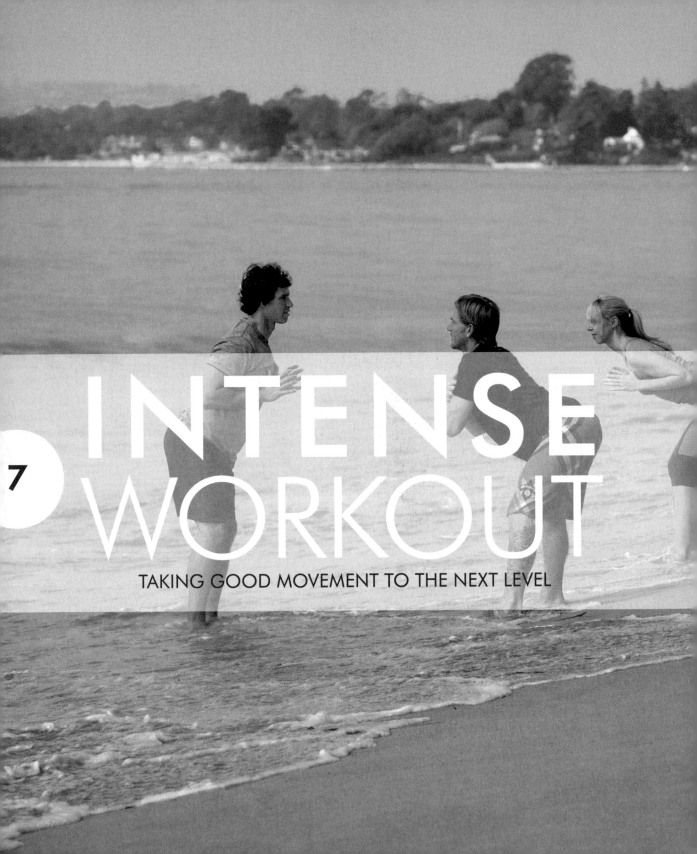

INTENSE WORKOUT

TAKING GOOD MOVEMENT TO THE NEXT LEVEL

7

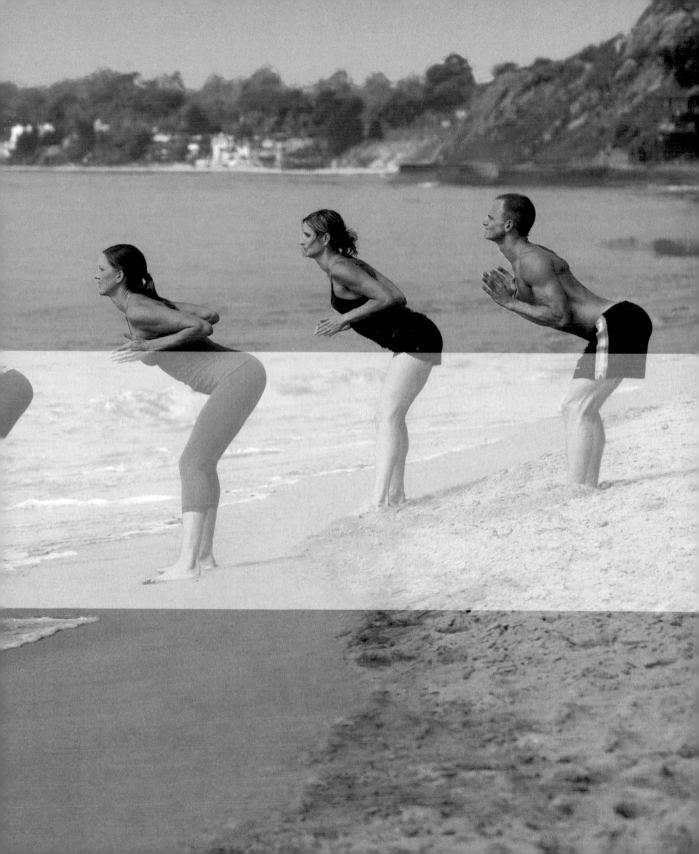

THE INTENSE WORKOUT AT A GLANCE

Repeat sequence three times to complete workout.

Time: 40 minutes

EXERCISE 1: THE FOUNDER

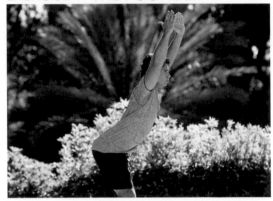

EXERCISE 2: FOUNDATION SQUAT

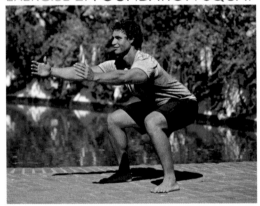

EXERCISE 3: GOOD MORNING

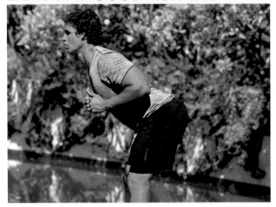

EXERCISE 4: WINDMILL

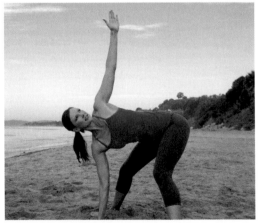

EXERCISE 5: WOODPECKER

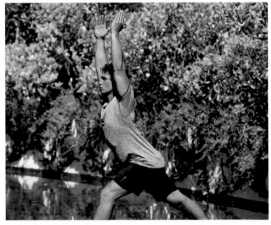

EXERCISE 6: BACK EXTENSION

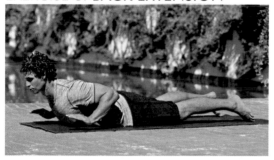

EXERCISE 7: FOUNDATION PLANK

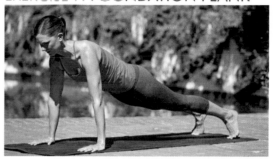

EXERCISE 8: ADDUCTOR-ASSISTED BACK EXTENSION

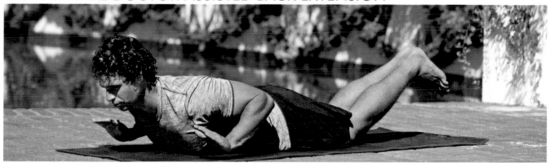

EXERCISE 9: CHILD'S POSE/ KNEELING FOUNDER

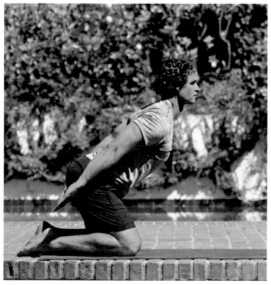

EXERCISE 10: LUNGE STRETCH

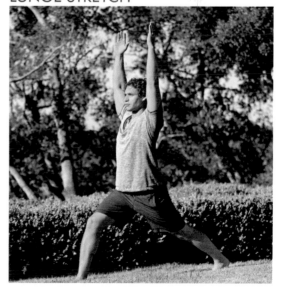

Though it may not have seemed possible a month ago, you have conquered pain or at least put it in its place. When our clients reach this stage, they are believers and are eager to see where Foundation training will take them. Most feel the best they have in years and want to keep it that way. Now that you are feeling this strong, it's time to take advantage of the renewed energy that comes from the physical and emotional relief of not having pain drag you down.

This intense 40-minute workout of 10 exercises will take you to the next level.

This workout is about power. At this stage, you will continue to strengthen your back in order to prevent injuries in the future, but the focus of the new movements is repetitive hinging power to train your body to keep your back extended. In the Intense Workout, you will circuit through these exercises three times.

After 6 weeks of progressively difficult exercises, Foundation training will be an important part of your life. No one we have worked with, including ourselves, has ever hit a plateau with Foundation training. Our clients tell us they are getting stronger each time they do a workout, and the same is true for both of us. There are endless variations to these essential exercises to make them more challenging. You can find some on our Web site, www.foundationroots.com; they will give you an idea of the direction Foundation can take you.

You may sometimes have back flare-ups, but after Foundation training, your body will be better able to cope with an injury. If back pain returns, simply cycle back to the basic or moderate workouts, depending on your level of pain.

When your body feels powerful, all sorts of physical activities open up to

> You can use these principles of movement to excel in other training methods and sports, from weight lifting to biking, from tennis to basketball.

you. You can use these principles of movement to excel in other training methods and sports, from weight lifting to biking, from tennis to basketball. *You* are in charge now, not your pain.

FOUNDATION FIRST

FROM SEVERE INJURY TO COMEBACK

I've never been tested quite as much as when I was hit by a car while riding my bike at 35 mph. I shattered my kneecap into three-"ish" pieces, and my professional cycling career was quickly put in jeopardy. It all happened so quickly, yet it took me months to wrap my head around the severity of my injury. I knew I was going to be able to walk again, but to ride again at the top level of the Pro Cycling peloton was at the forefront of my concern.

Not one to wallow in self-pity, I turned my negative situation into a positive one. I began assembling a formidable team of some of the best physical therapists, chiropractors, acupuncturists, and health practitioners I could find to help me return to cycling stronger and faster than I had been before. I set off on a mission. Once I committed myself, the doors began to open. In December 2009, almost 7 months after my accident, I discovered Peter Park and Eric Goodman at the Platinum Fitness Studio in Santa Barbara. These two men were the keystone to my recovery. They gave me Foundation training and gave me my career back.

The Foundation exercises increased my strength, flexibility, coordination, and balance more rapidly than I ever could have imagined. I went from having a hard time walking up and down stairs in late December 2009 to competing in the Amgen Tour of California in May 2010. This is the largest cycling event in North America and attracts some of the best cyclists around the globe. I was not only able to meet my goal of finishing the 7-day, 812-mile race, but I was also able to finish inside the top 20 and be highly competitive day in and day out.

Since then, I have taken these exercises to heart and put them in my training regimen year-round. They helped get me back to racing competitively as well as cured other imbalances I had developed after years of racing my bike and neglecting my core strength. I encourage everyone to have the open mind I did when seeking help for my injury. Follow that path and a better, healthier lifestyle is right around the corner.

LUCAS EUSER, PROFESSIONAL CYCLIST

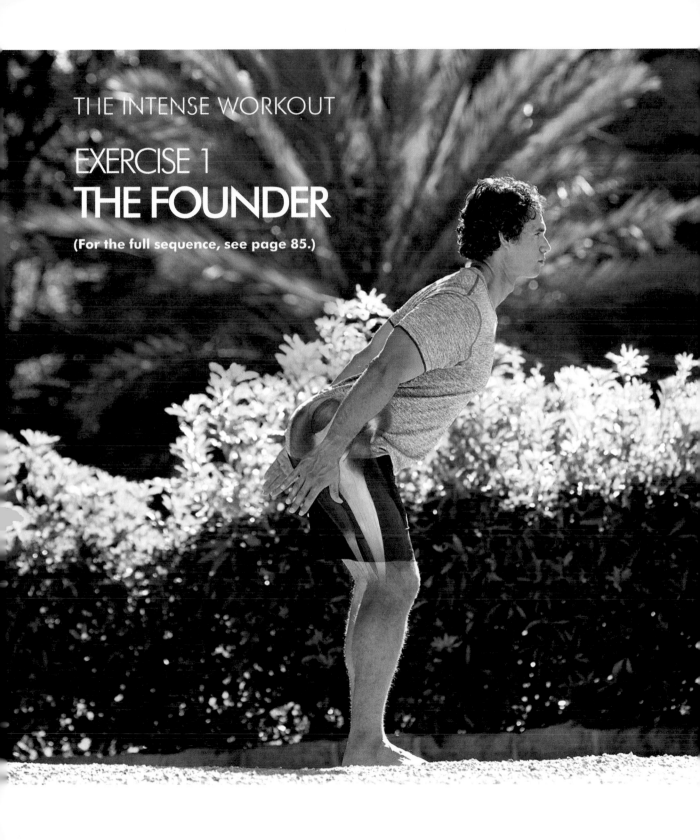

THE INTENSE WORKOUT

EXERCISE 1
THE FOUNDER

(For the full sequence, see page 85.)

EXERCISE 2
FOUNDATION SQUAT (20 REPS)

Increase to 20 reps and try to go lower. (For the full sequence, see page 116.)

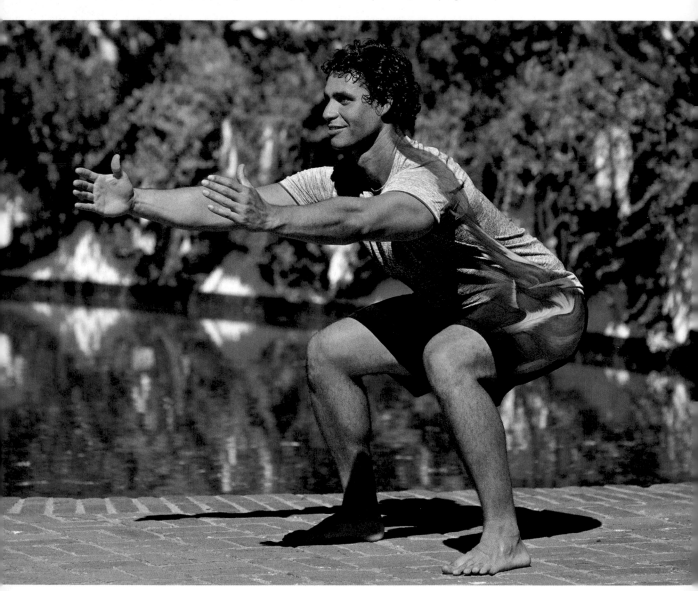

EXERCISE 3
GOOD MORNING (15 REPS)

This exercise emphasizes the all-important hinge. The Good Morning trains your body to move gracefully and forcefully from the hip joints, without any force on the spine. Focus on stretching down and contracting the same muscle groups. Once you learn this movement pattern, your life will begin to change.

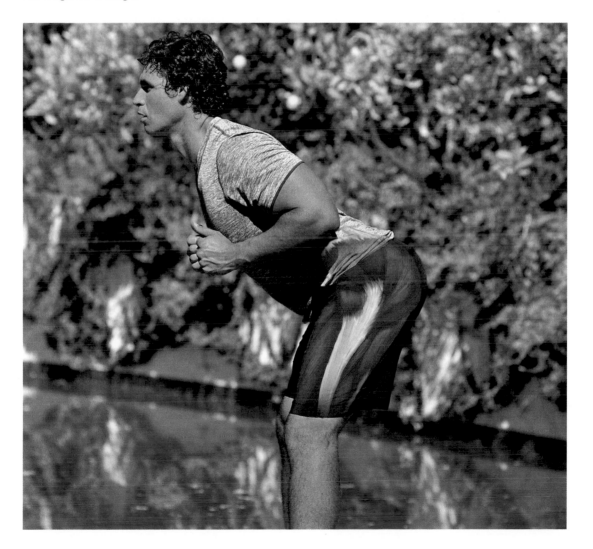

GOOD MORNING

Working the glutes and hamstrings, this exercise is the hinge maker.

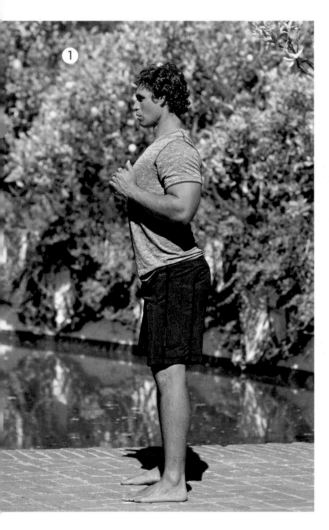 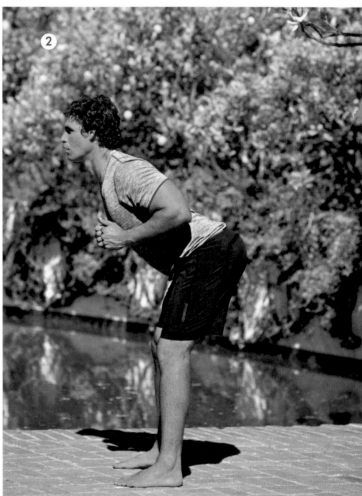

1 With feet shoulder-width apart and arms across your chest, start pressing your butt behind you.

2 Hinge forward at the hips, keeping your chest up and back straight. Do not allow your spine to flex forward. Your knees should be slightly bent and your weight should be fully on your heels.

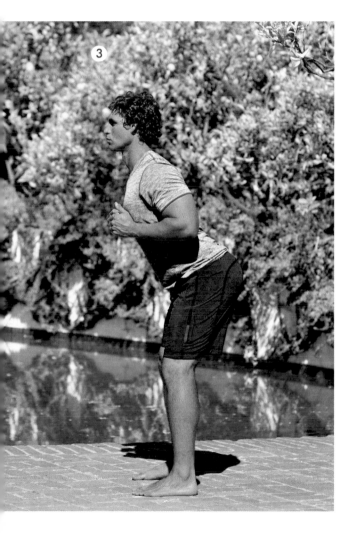 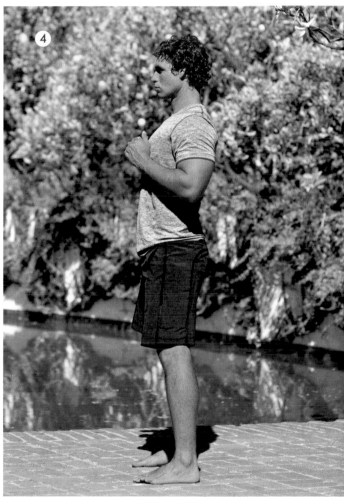

3 Keep your spine extended and your chest held up high, and pull yourself quickly back up, using your glutes and hamstrings.

4 Contract your butt muscles all the way up to the top of the movement, and repeat 14 times.

THE PERFECT GOOD MORNING

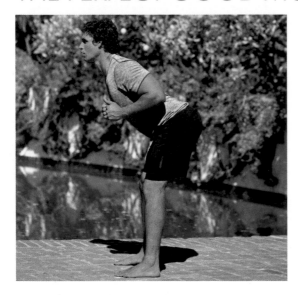

The right motion recruits your glutes and hamstrings. To do that, you have to:

- Hinge at hips.
- Hold chest high, with back extended.
- Bend knees slightly for full power of hamstrings.
- Keep weight on heels.
- Contract glutes to pull up torso.

TROUBLESHOOTING THE GOOD MORNING

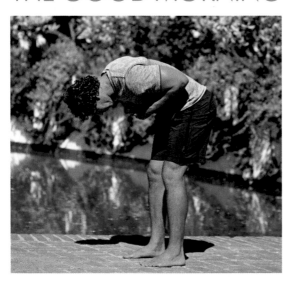

- Hinge from flexed spine.
- Shoulders are raised.
- Knees are straight.
- Weight is forward on toes.
- Torso pulls up from lumbar spine, vertebra by vertebra.

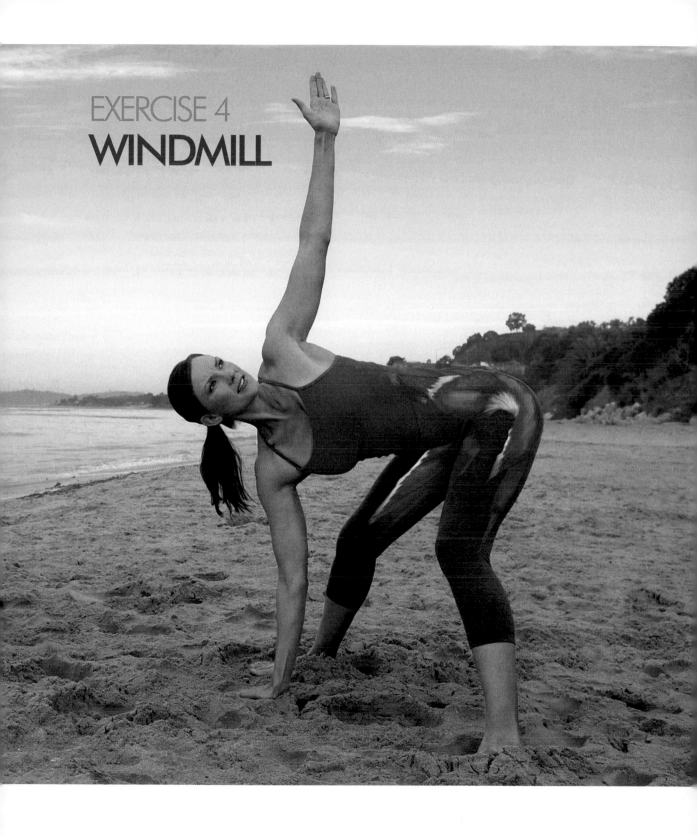

EXERCISE 4
WINDMILL

WINDMILL

This exercise is used to create a deep, active stretch at the upper adductor muscles, the inner thighs. These muscles are a strong anchor on the pelvis. They pull hard and can significantly affect your lower-spine movement when tight. If you spend a lot of time sitting, this exercise is a perfect antidote.

The primary stretch in this exercise is at the upper adductor. As in all Foundation exercises, other muscles are involved, in this instance a full sweep: the erector spinae, hamstrings, glutes, and quadratus lumborum.

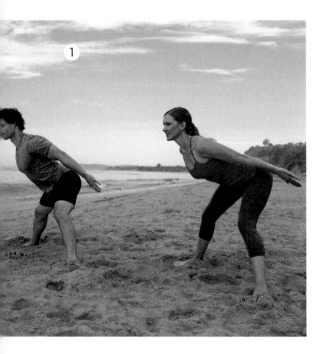 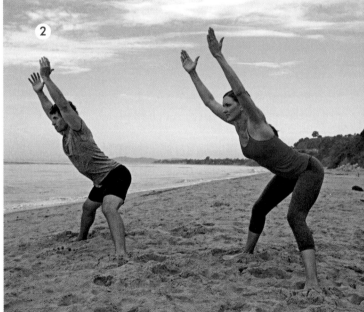

① Start in a very wide-legged Founder position, legs slightly bent and hips pushed back, with your weight on your heels. Bring your arms out in front of you and hold for 15 seconds.

② Raise your arms, keeping your weight on your heels and your shoulders pulled down your back.

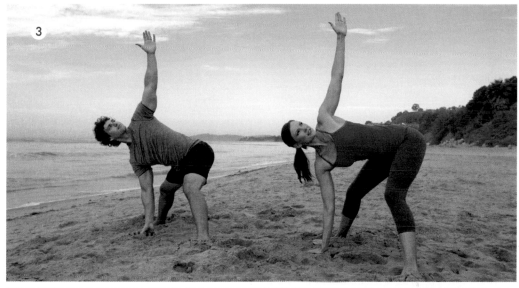

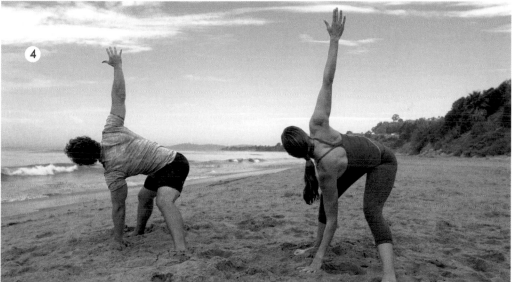

3 Keeping your shoulders back and your back flat with your knees slightly bent, fold forward, bringing your right arm down to the ground below your chest. Rotate your left arm as high as you can in a twist. The hardest part is keeping your pelvis squared. Make sure both knees are bent, and keep your weight back on the heels. Hold for 20 to 30 seconds.

4 Switch by bringing your left arm to the floor, pulling your weight farther back on the heels and switching arms. Rotate your right arm as high as you can in a twist. Hold for 20 to 30 seconds.

THE PERFECT WINDMILL

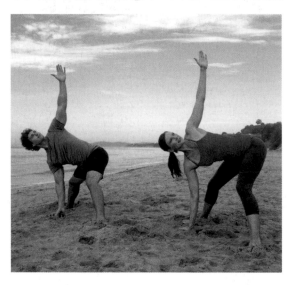

- Hinge from hips.
- Extend your back.
- Spread legs far apart.
- Keep pelvis squared.
- Keep knees slightly bent.
- Place weight on heels.

TROUBLESHOOTING THE WINDMILL

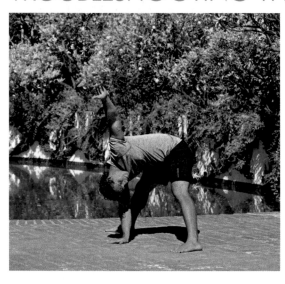

- Bend is from lower back with a flexed spine.
- Legs are too close together for good balance.
- Pelvis tilts forward.
- Knees are straight.
- Weight is shifted forward.

EXERCISE 5
WOODPECKER

Try to get a strong contraction on each movement. (For the full sequence, see page 121.)

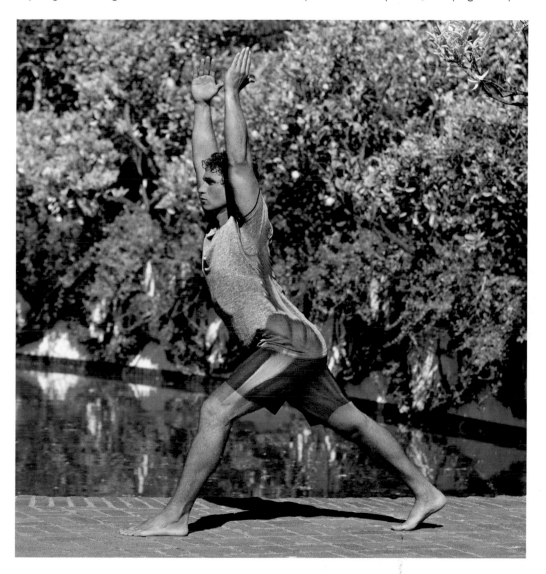

EXERCISE 6
BACK EXTENSION (20 REPS)

(For the full sequence, see page 91.)

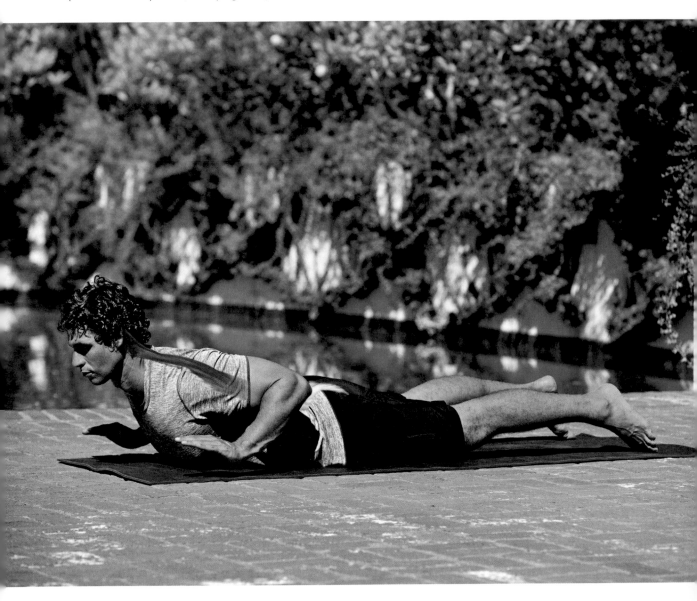

EXERCISE 7
FOUNDATION PLANK

A plank with a difference, the Foundation version of the standard plank goes deeper, working the deep abdominal muscles, rectus abdominus, multifidi, and iliopsoas.

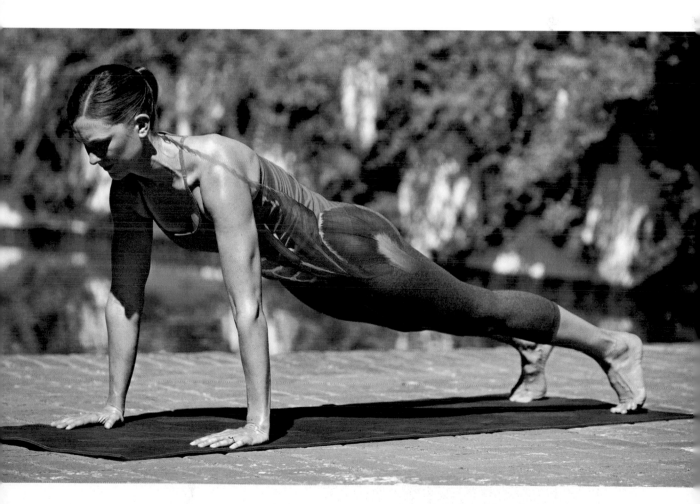

FOUNDATION PLANK

The Foundation variation on a conventional plank will get to a far deeper part of the abs and hips. This is done by changing the angles and weight distribution throughout the movement. We use the Foundation Plank to build pelvic stability and train the hips to move independently of the spine.

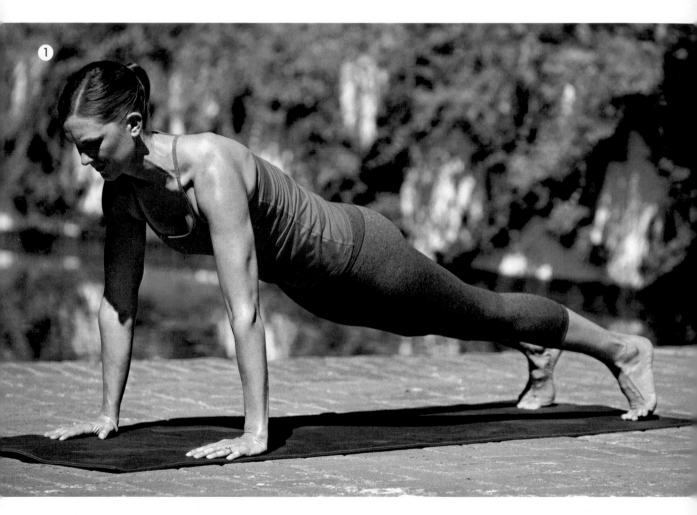

1 Press up to a rigid plank, a high pushup position. Keep your body in a straight line. Do not drop your hips. Your weight is on your toes.

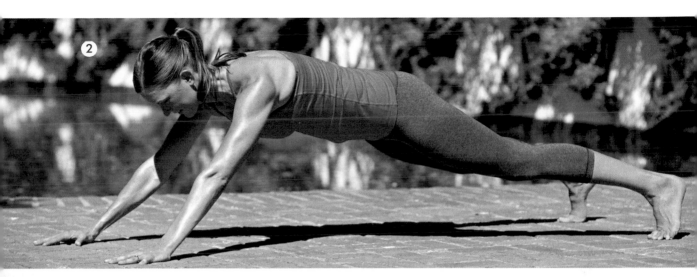

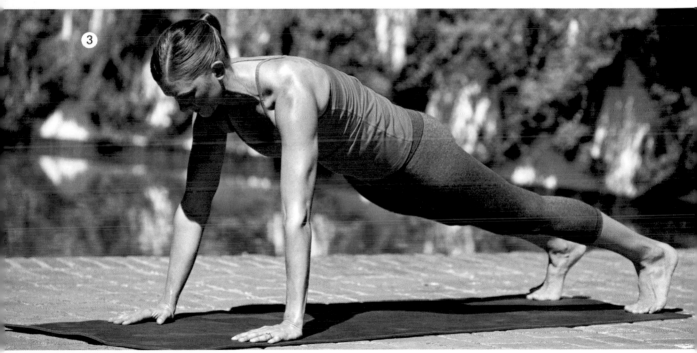

② Slowly walk your arms forward 6 inches. Press your heels down as far as you can. Drop your hips about 2 inches. Hold for 30 seconds.

③ Slowly walk your arms back directly under your shoulders.

THE PERFECT FOUNDATION PLANK

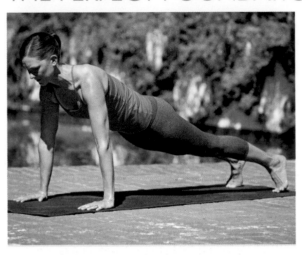

- A perfect plank forms a rigid line from the ears to the heels.
- Shoulders are tight, stomach is braced, glutes and quads are tight.
- Arms are strong, and hands and fingers are spread out open on the floor. We even want to focus on wrist strength.

TROUBLESHOOTING THE FOUNDATION PLANK

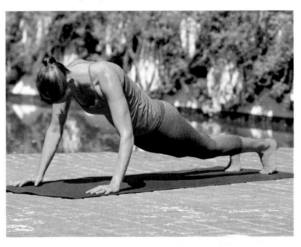

- Line sags, with stomach dropped.
- Arms are bent.

EXERCISE 8
ADDUCTOR-ASSISTED BACK EXTENSION
(20- TO 30-SECOND HOLDS)

Squeezing your knees makes this exercise effective. (For the full sequence, see page 95.)

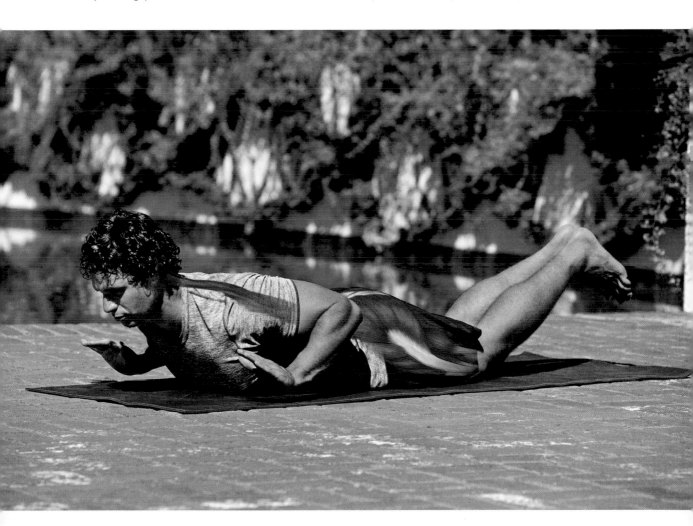

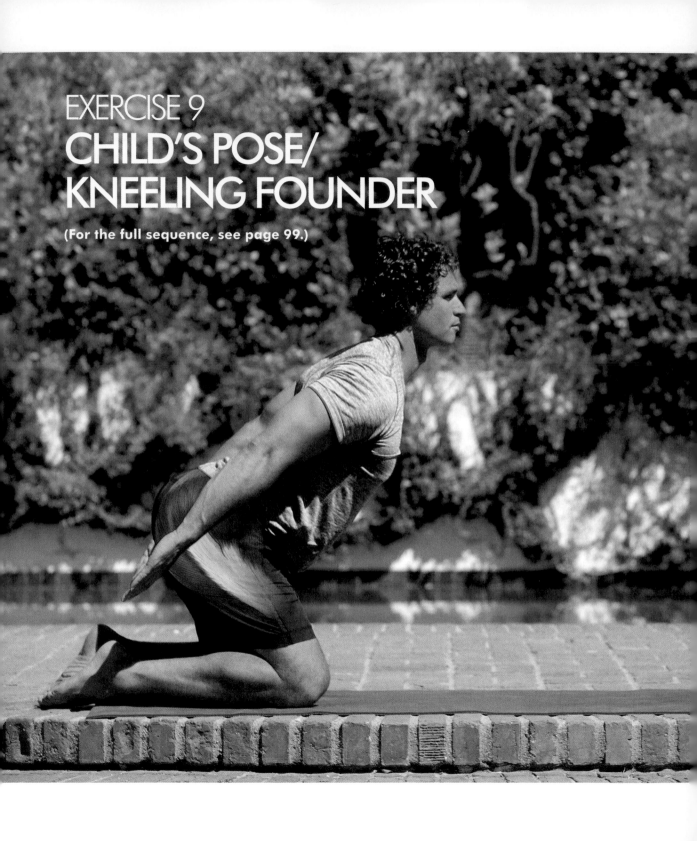

EXERCISE 9
CHILD'S POSE/ KNEELING FOUNDER

(For the full sequence, see page 99.)

EXERCISE 10
LUNGE STRETCH
(HOLD 30 SECONDS PER SIDE)

(For the full sequence, see page 104.)

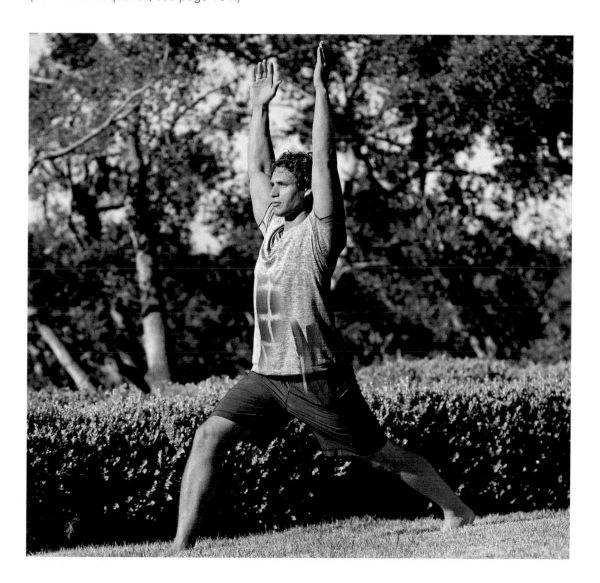

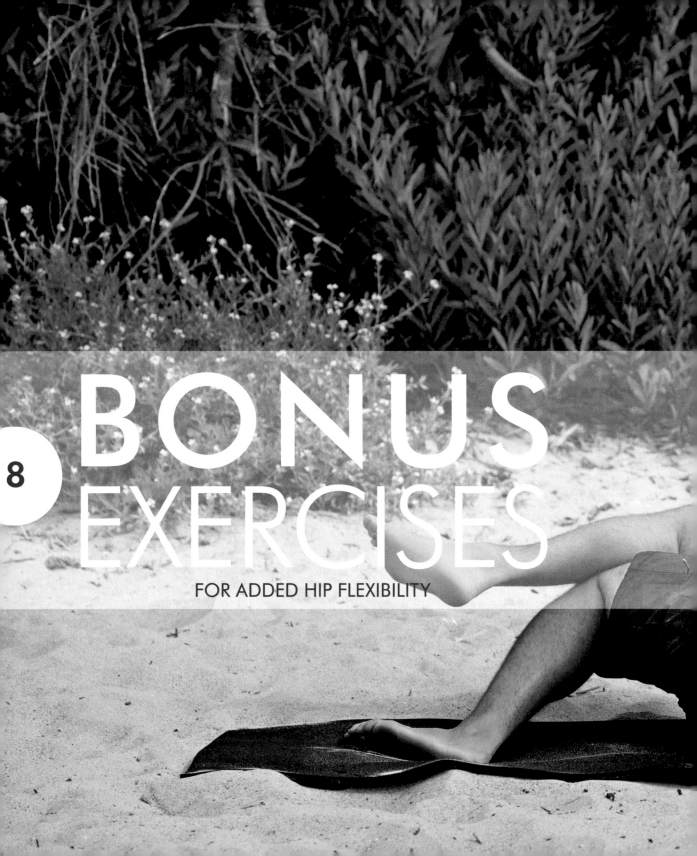

BONUS EXERCISES

FOR ADDED HIP FLEXIBILITY

8

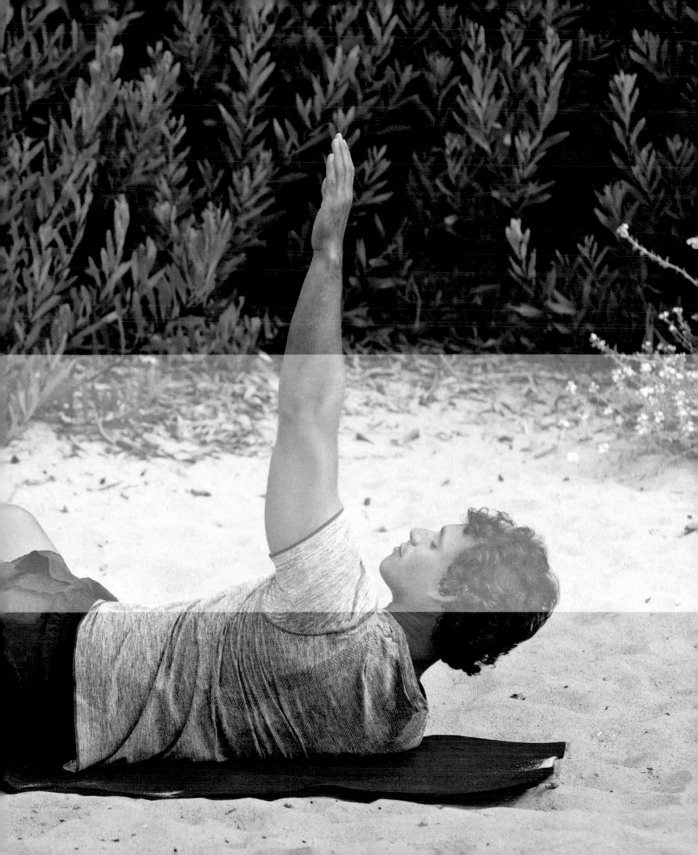

THE
HIP
WORKOUT
AT A GLANCE

BONUS EXERCISE 1: **CROSSOVER**

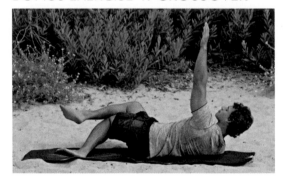

BONUS EXERCISE 2: **CROSS UNDER**

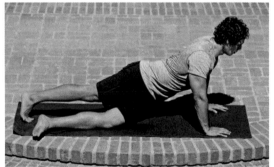

ip pain is so common because we spend so much time sitting. Sitting causes your hip muscles to contract, and they need to be stretched for you to have ease of movement. In modern life, our hip flexors are not extended most of the time, and this problem is only compounded by age—as we get older, our muscles tighten up more. Think of how children can sit on the floor with their legs crossed in front of them for hours, how easily they bend, and how flexible they are. How long has it been since you were able to sit in the lotus position? Or bend effortlessly? Or do a squat without feeling creaky?

If you have hip pain, you are probably well aware of it, but one way to test how tight your hip muscles and joints are is to sit with a straight back on the edge of a chair with one leg crossed over the other. If the knee of your crossed leg is approximately level with your lower leg when you are relaxed in the position, your hip muscles are in good shape. The higher your crossed knee is, the tighter

Hip pain is a complex issue with many potential causes. You can experience hip pain when resting, when moving, or when standing for very different reasons. If hip pain is persistent, you should see a doctor for a diagnosis.

your hip joint is. Check both legs to see which side is tighter than the other.

If too much sitting and bad posture are responsible for your hip pain, these bonus exercises will help release tension and stiffness by relaxing your pelvis muscles. Relaxing these muscles allows the pelvis to move naturally in squatting and bending, relieving most tension from the outer hip.

The hip stretches in this chapter can be done as additions to the Foundation workout or separately. These simple exercises can make a tangible change in your flexibility. They take less than 10 minutes a day and deliver fast results.

FOUNDATIONFIRST

The Foundation work I've been doing with Peter Park has been a perfect complement to my core strength training. The results have given me greater strength, coordination, and balance. As a cyclist, I am much more flexible and relaxed on the bike, have increased my stem length, and can ride miles in the drops without any neck or back discomfort. In my opinion, Foundation is essential to any fitness or athletic training program.

JIM THOMAS

THE HIP WORKOUT

BONUS EXERCISE 1
CROSSOVER

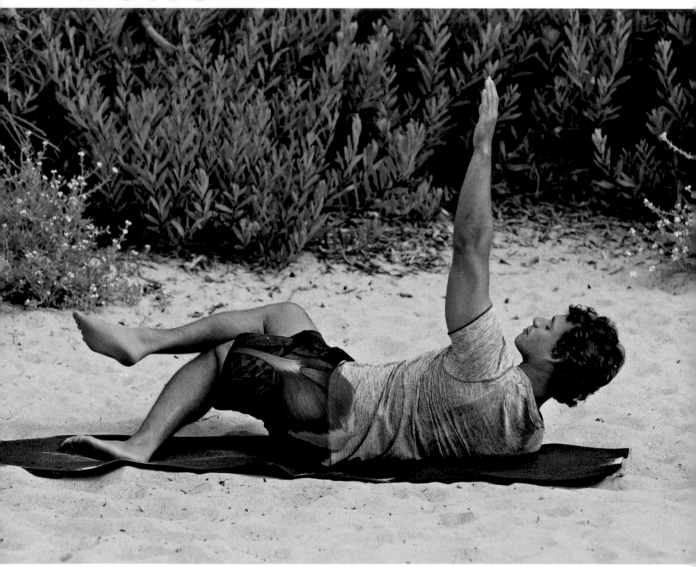

CROSSOVER

One of the most important muscles in the pelvis is the iliacus muscle, which lines the inner border of the pelvis and is responsible for pelvic contraction and relaxation. The more the pelvis moves with bending and squatting, the easier overall movement becomes. This exercise stretches the iliacus muscle, along with the psoas, IT band, and several muscles in the torso.

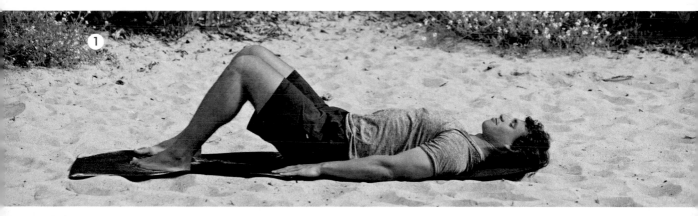

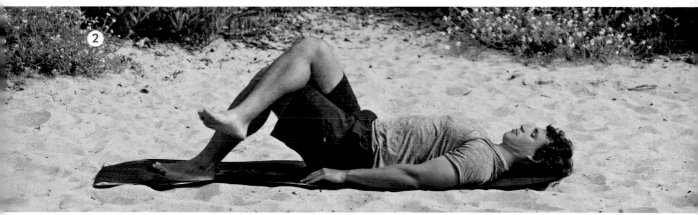

1 Lie on your back with your knees bent and your feet flat on the floor about 2 feet in front of your butt. Your arms should be resting by your sides.

2 Cross your right leg over the left and keep your knees very close together.

If you have knee pain while doing this exercise, we suggest you skip it.

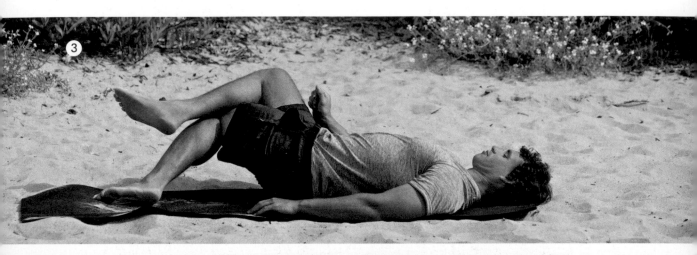

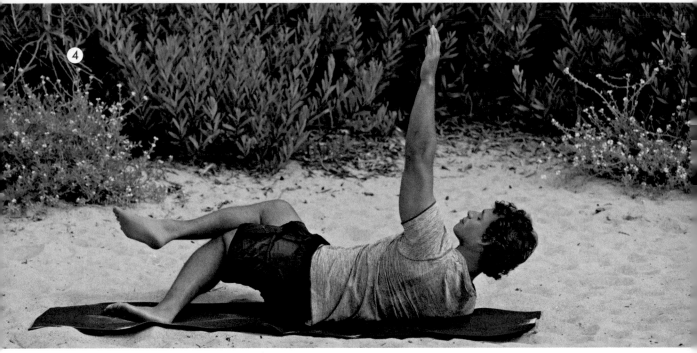

3 Using your right leg as a lever, pull your left knee all the way across your body to the ground. Bring your left arm all the way back over your head and breathe as deeply as you can. Feel the stretch in your upper left hip.

4 Raise your left arm in the air and crunch straight up 5 to 10 times.

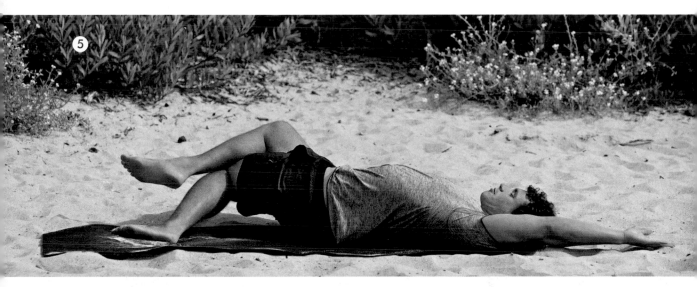

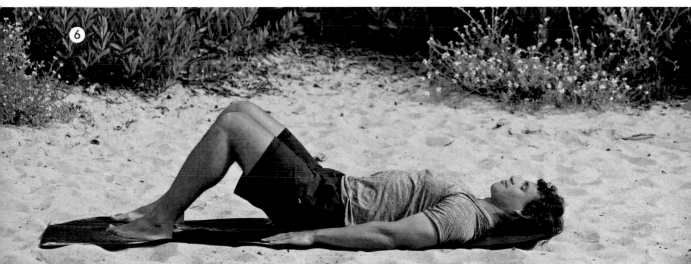

⑤ Bring your left arm back behind you and stretch further for 15 seconds before switching sides.

⑥ Return to the starting position and switch sides.

THE PERFECT CROSSOVER

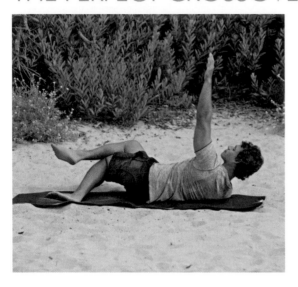

- Knees should be crossed as close together as possible, with both legs bent a bit more than 90 degrees.
- The stretch is felt through the hip, abs, and leg on the side that is up off the ground.
- Reaching the arm overhead and behind creates a deeper, longer stretch along that same leg.

TROUBLESHOOTING THE CROSSOVER

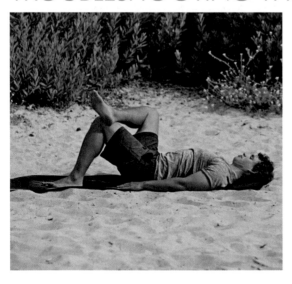

- Knees are not crossed close together.
- There's not enough stretching overhead.

BONUS EXERCISE 2
CROSS UNDER

This exercises the IT band, which goes from the lower midspine to the pelvis, hip flexors, and quadratus lumborum. The stretch should be felt along the leg on the bottom in the hip, IT band, and above the hip into the oblique muscles.

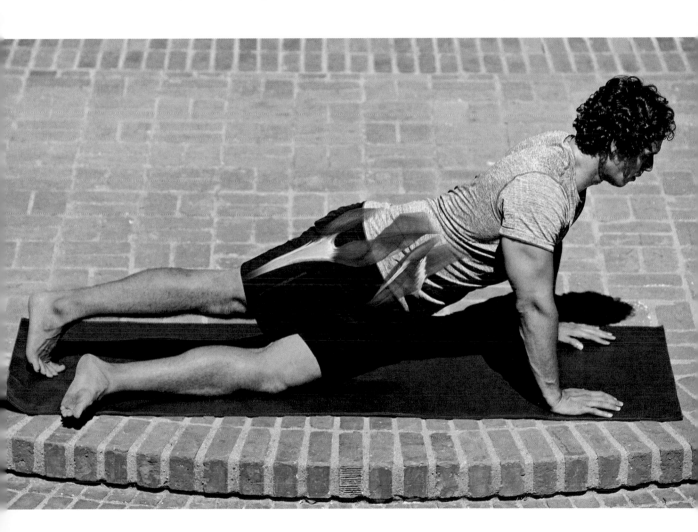

CROSS UNDER

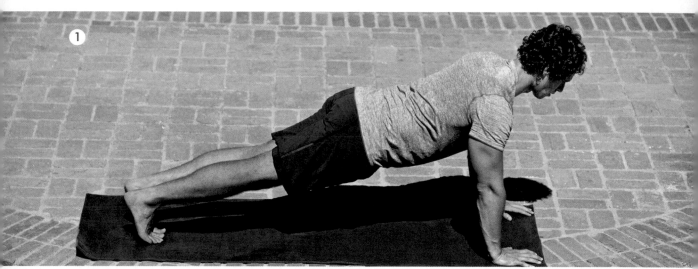

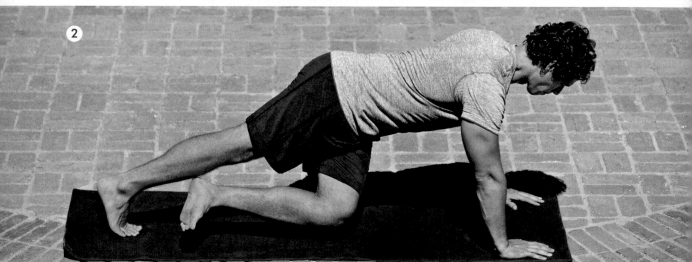

If this stretch feels as if it is pinching the lower back on the side of the straight leg, we suggest you skip it.

1 Press yourself into a rigid plank/high pushup.

2 Bring your left leg underneath your right and let your left knee bend slightly.

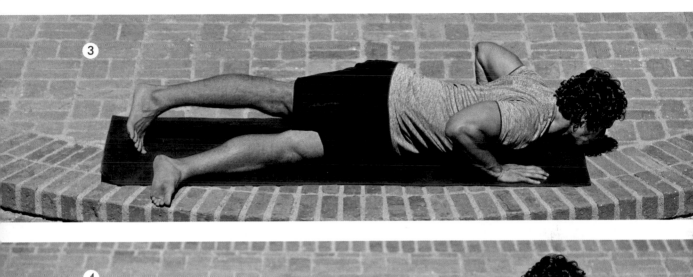

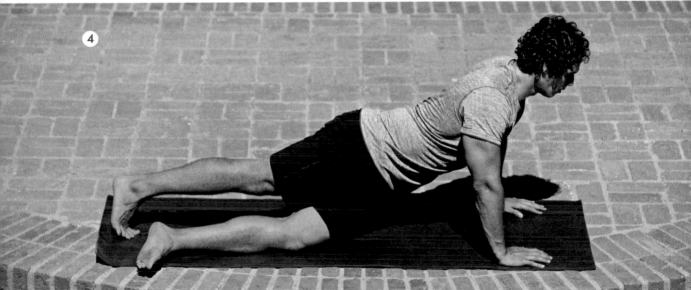

3 Slowly lower yourself down onto your left hip. Walk your hands forward a few inches and square up your shoulders.

4 Keeping your hips on the floor, push your chest up and pull it forward. Keep your head up and pulled away from your shoulders. Rotate your right heel up to help square your hips. You should feel this stretch along the left side of your body, along the lower leg in the hip, in the IT band, and above the hip into the oblique muscles. Hold for 20 seconds.

Repeat on the other side.

THE PERFECT CROSS UNDER

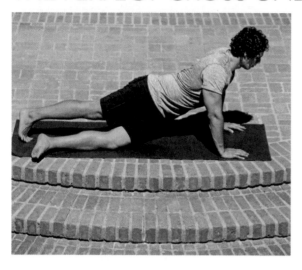

- The Cross Under is tricky—when done correctly, feet are only 1 to 1½ feet apart.
- Shoulders should be squared in front and arms should shake a little while chest is pressed up.

TROUBLESHOOTING THE CROSS UNDER

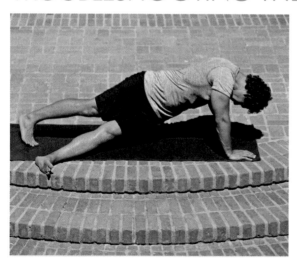

- Feet are too far apart after the Cross Under.
- Torso is turned.

The exercises you have learned in these chapters will take you a long way toward achieving flexibility, endurance, and power. Foundation training has to become a part of your life if you want the movement to carry over into everything you do. Do not stop doing these workouts when you feel better. That is an invitation for your back problems to return.

These exercises can do so much more for you than to "fix" a back problem.

Since you feel so good, we also want you to pay more attention to the care and feeding of your body. Our clients have started to feel so good that they've gone on to transfer their new fitness to all aspects of their life. We call it the Foundation lifestyle. Keep reading, and we will show you how to support your progress with diet, sleep, relaxation, and balanced physical activity.

> Do not stop doing these workouts when you feel better. That is an invitation for your back problems to return. These exercises can do so much more for you than to "fix" a back problem.

9

THE FOUNDATION LIFESTYLE

INTEGRATING FOUNDATION PRINCIPLES INTO YOUR EVERYDAY LIFE

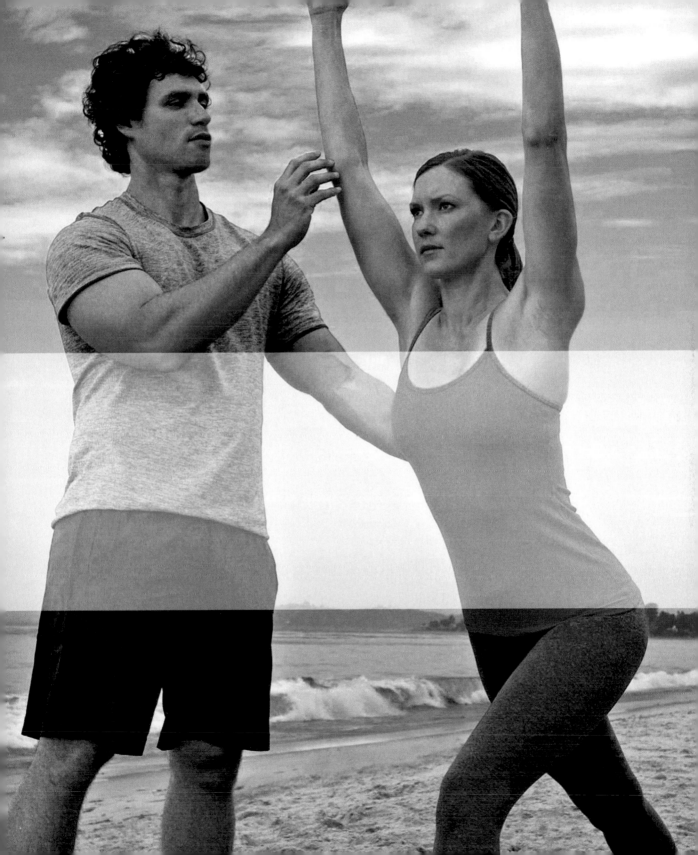

Being in pain takes a lot of energy. Just doing everyday things like getting out of bed in the morning, tying your shoelaces, lowering yourself into the seat of your car, getting up from your desk, carrying a grocery bag, or even picking up your 2-year-old requires such effort. Back pain saps the energy out of you, making you cranky and generally exhausted. As you break through the barriers that pain has created in your life, you are going to feel your energy and power return. And as you begin to feel better and do so much more, the Foundation perspective will inform everything else in your life. You have only one body, and you'll want to treat yours better

> As you break through the barriers that pain has created in your life, you are going to feel your energy and power return.

once you see how the small changes you've made in your life have taken you from pain to performance.

You might have been able to get away with bad habits when you were in your twenties, but as you get older, lifestyle factors take a toll on your body. Poor eating habits, excessive alcohol consumption, and lack of sleep begin to show themselves once you get to your forties and fifties. We think of the megasuccessful business-people we've encountered. If they are not sitting at a desk all day long, they are on an airplane. They travel around the world for meetings and conferences, get jet-lagged, and lose sleep. Entertaining is an important aspect of their professional lives, and consuming rich food and alcohol is almost part of the job description. By the time they are in their forties or fifties, they are tight and immobile. The way they live and the pressures of their jobs are visible on their skin. We've trained people like this. The Foundation lifestyle has made a substantial difference in the way they feel, and we can see how much better they look.

SUPPLEMENTS FOR THE RELIEF OF BACK PAIN

Many natural remedies can help with pain relief. This is a short list of our favorites. The natural remedy market is largely unregulated. Do not buy cheap supplements from your local drug store or supermarket. Go to a health food store or natural remedy pharmacy and ask questions. None of these will work miracles, but they can make your efforts far more effective.

Vitamin B_{12} is important for overall nervous system function. Sublingual, or under the tongue, lozenges are best next to injections.

Vitamin D_3 has been shown to improve symptoms of back pain in numerous studies. Common dose recommendations are too low for significant effects. We recommend a daily dose between 4,000 and 10,000 IU.

Magnesium supports healthy muscle and nerve function, keeps your heart rhythm steady, and supports overall immune system function.

Omega-3 fatty acids are strong anti-inflammatories but not in the frequently low recommended dosage. We recommend staying between 2,000 and 6,000 milligrams daily.

Glucosamine and chondroitin are important for the proper repair of connective tissue.

IF THERE WEREN'T ENOUGH REASONS NOT TO SMOKE . . .

Studies have shown that smoking cigarettes doubles the risk of suffering from severe back pain, because smoking affects circulation and reduces the blood supply to your muscles and bones. Smoking is a leading risk factor in degenerative disc disease. If you smoke, you are much more likely to have severe degeneration of your discs. From a mechanical point of view, the coughing that accompanies smoking also increases pressure and strain on your spine.

In addition to encouraging people to master the exercises at the core of Foundation training, we recommend an anti-inflammatory lifestyle, one that includes relaxation, restorative sleep, a metabolic tune-up, clean food, and exercise. Being overweight, obese, or in poor physical condition contributes to back pain, and each situation is entirely under your control.

You make choices in your life, and we promise you that when you are feeling good, it is easier to select healthier options. In this chapter, you will learn how you to make the right choices, and we'll provide you with a realistic plan for changing a toxic lifestyle.

STRESS, SLEEP, AND YOUR BACK

There is a very real connection between mental and physical pain; emotional stress has a lingering effect on your body. Your body holds emotional stress in your muscles. The tension in your muscles can compress blood vessels, reducing blood flow to the tissue. Your blood carries oxygen and nutrients to your muscles, bones, and joints. Without enough oxygen, your muscles can go into spasm. Depriving your muscles of nutrients may cause them to weaken. Just as there is a correlation between sedentary work and back pain, a stressful job can also increase your chance of developing back problems.

Stress hormones—cortisol in particular—heighten inflammation in the body. Constant stress can create chronic elevation of cortisol levels and make your nervous system hyperactive. Aside from leading to adrenal burnout, long-term overproduction of cortisol can disrupt your sleep and contribute to fat accumulation in your

L-THEANINE FOR NATURAL STRESS RELIEF

We don't recommend taking many supplements, because they are costly and often entirely ineffective, but we have seen what this natural anxiety reducer and mood enhancer can do. L-theanine, found in green tea leaves, is an amino acid that is able to cross the blood-brain barrier and improve your brain's reaction to stress. It has been shown to reduce mental and physical stress while sharpening thinking and improving mood. L-theanine stimulates the production of alpha brain waves, creating a state of deep relaxation and mental alertness similar to what is achieved through meditation. L-theanine also affects the balance of dopamine and serotonin in the brain to create a relaxation effect.

You can find L-theanine supplements in any health food store. It's not a bad idea to add green tea to your diet, too.

abdomen, which is guaranteed to make your back muscles work harder. Cortisol is a metabolic nemesis because it promotes the storage of what you eat as fat.

Stress can stimulate so many different unhealthy behaviors—smoking, excessive consumption of alcohol or caffeine, bad eating habits, and sleep disorders, to name a few. To incorporate the Foundation lifestyle into your life, begin by building in time to relax each day. If you find yourself grinding your teeth or your shoulders are rising up to your ears, take a minute to breathe deeply—slowly inhale and exhale from your belly. The tension will melt from your body, and your mind will calm down. As you have seen, we use deep breathing in Foundation workouts to ensure your muscles have adequate oxygen and nutrients to work with maximum efficiency and power.

Meditation has been proven to be an effective tool for mental and physical relaxation. Everyone we have met who meditates claims significant benefits. The idea is to clear your mind of the constant inner monologue. The directed focus of the Foundation workout, done slowly and in a mindful way, can be a form of meditation in and of itself. If you concentrate on your Foundation exercises, you will increase the benefit physically and mentally.

R&R

Things happen at breakneck speed in this day and age, and as a rule, people are trying to get by with less and less sleep. Some of our clients say, "Oh, I can get by on 4½ or 5 hours of sleep." Maybe they think they are doing fine, but they don't realize what zombies they are until they actually get enough restful shut-eye.

You need 7 or 8 hours of sleep a night so that your body can recover and regenerate. Exactly how much sleep you need depends on your age (the younger you are, the more you need—think of how long a baby sleeps), what you do when you are awake, and your genes. If you are training for a triathlon, you will need more sleep than someone who sits at a desk 8 hours a day and watches TV all night.

If you try to get by on less than 7 or 8 hours, you will pay for it in ways you might not expect. Sleep is not a passive state. A lot goes on in your body while you are getting some shut-eye. Your brain organizes and solidifies learning and memory, which improves your concentration and promotes innovative and flexible thinking. Sleep strengthens your immune system and allows repair in your nervous system. Growth hormone is released during sleep to repair muscle tissue. Deep sleep relieves stress by quieting your aroused nervous system. The production of cortisol is at its lowest when you sleep. A good night's sleep will regulate your mood as well.

Inadequate sleep leads to weight gain. There is a direct correlation between the obesity epidemic, the rise of sleep disorders, and the trend toward fewer hours of sleep each night. Here's how it works: The appetite-suppressant hormone is produced while you sleep, and if you don't get enough sleep or it's of poor quality, the delicate balance of your hormones goes out of whack and appetite-stimulating hormones dominate, making you hungrier all day long.

Sleep deprivation is a serious matter, and it goes beyond the simple "brain fog" you may experience after a night of tossing and turning. There are a number of signs that indicate you are sleep deprived. You need to change your habits and get more sleep if:

- You need to nap often.

- You nod off for very brief periods during the day.

- You fall asleep the minute your head hits the pillow.

- You need an alarm clock to wake you.

The amount of time you sleep is as important as the hours that you are awake. Sleep pays a high dividend. Don't shortchange yourself.

METABOLIC TUNE-UP

After breaking through your back pain, you will probably be ready for a metabolic tune-up to get your body into great shape. Whether we suffer from chronic pain or not, most of us can afford to lose a few pounds. Sedentary lifestyles and bad eating habits have led to a global weight problem. If you've been sidelined by pain, the likelihood that you've put on a few pounds is even higher.

The goal of this tune-up is to burn as many calories as you can while maintaining muscle development and strength. You can create a long-term increase in your metabolic rate without drugs, weight loss pills, or energy drinks.

Here's how. For starters, you have to be realistic and acknowledge that you, like everyone else, have a baseline metabolism that creates a template from which you must work. You are born with a genetic code that directs your body to operate at a comfortable pace, called a set point. If you are born a pickup truck, chances are that no matter what you do, achieving the efficiency of a Prius is not in your future. On the other hand, if you make smart choices, you can become one of those hybrid trucks that show some improvement in efficiency.

You have control of about 10 to 15 percent of your metabolism through natural means. This increase many not sound impressive, but let's look at the numbers. If you are naturally burning 3,000 calories a day, a 10 percent increase of 300 calories a day adds up to 109,500 additional calories burned in a year. With no other factors present, this increase can translate to more than 30 pounds of lost weight in a year. If you throw in the additional exercise we are going to recommend, there is no limit to how you can burn toxic fat, strengthen your muscles, and take undue stress off your back.

EAT TO LIVE, DON'T LIVE TO EAT

Changing what and how much you eat is a big shift in lifestyle, one that is essential to your health and well-being. One way to begin is to stop thinking of food as a reward. Food is fuel. The better you eat, the better your body will run. If you had a Ferrari, would you use the cheapest gas you could find? If you did, your fine-tuned machine would have serious mechanical problems, and the car would be in the shop

KEEP TRACK OF WHAT YOU PUT IN YOUR MOUTH

Keeping a food log will give you an accurate picture of how you are fueling your body. You cannot be in great shape if your body isn't getting adequate nourishment for energy and optimal functioning of its interacting systems.

Here's rule number one of the food log: Don't cheat. If you are going to change the way you eat, you have to be realistic about how far you have to go to replace bad eating habits with good ones.

You can carry a notebook or index cards with you so that you *immediately* write down what you are eating. That way you won't end up trying to reconstruct exactly what it was that you scarfed down on your way to your morning meeting. You can use a phone app or one of the many free food tracker Web sites. Those tools not only provide calorie counts but also analyze the composition of what you eat in terms of protein, carbohydrates, fats, and sugar. They will show you how much of your caloric goal you have consumed and whether you are meeting the nutritional requirements of your body. You can adapt the settings to your individual activity levels and calorie requirements.

We like the food log on the LIVESTRONG Web site (also available as an app) called My Plate. You can access My Plate in two ways:

www.livestrong.com (Log on to My Plate from the home page.)

www.thedailyplate.com (This address is for direct access to the food log on LIVESTRONG.)

every other week. The same is true for your body. If you feed it sugar and chemicals, it will break down.

Whenever we take on new clients, we have them complete a food log to make them aware of how much they are really eating. The reaction after a week is always "I can't believe there are thousands of extra calories I didn't know about!" The bite of your kid's breakfast, the cookie, that handful of cashews you eat without thinking—it all adds up. You have to be conscious of what you are eating, and you have to make a commitment to do better.

NO MORE MONSTER PORTIONS

Peter had a rude awakening when he traveled to Europe to race. At lunch or dinner, he would look at the size of the portion on his plate and think, *Are you kidding me? You call that a meal?* His expectations were skewed from living in the United States his whole life, where bigger is better. There are some restaurants in this country that give portions large enough to feed three people. Peter realized the European portions were the way to go. It was time for him to get real about serving sizes.

When we eat more than we need, all those calories that don't burn off get stored as fat. You should train yourself to think, *Okay, have I had enough food here?* You have to think about *why* you are eating. Most important, you have to control the serving size of the food you eat, eat your food slowly, and enjoy it. Know when to push that stop button.

Base your portions on how active you are. If you sit at a desk all day and exercise 20 or 30 minutes a week, or if you are traveling, you do not need to eat much—maybe 1,500 to 1,800 calories a day. You have to eat lightly and avoid simple carbohydrates like bread and pasta. If you are going on a 4-hour hike, you will need to eat more and consume some carbs for energy. Your carbohydrate intake and portion size depend on your output—that is, what you are doing.

There are a number of tricks to help you control your portion size.

• Think of a full plate. Now take a quarter of that away. The resulting portion is the amount of food you should be eating at each meal. Making that small change alone could help you lose a pound of weight in a week.

• Studies have shown that if you eat from a smaller plate, your brain perceives the portion to be larger and thinks you are eating more than you actually consume. The result is that you get full on less food. So eat from a salad plate instead of a dinner plate. Your smaller portions won't look lost on a big, almost empty dish.

• If you are going out to eat, you don't have to eat everything on your plate. Ask for a doggie bag. It's great to have leftovers in the fridge for another meal.

• If you are starving before going out to eat or to a party, eat a few almonds or an apple before you leave home. A healthy snack will curb your appetite.

• If you find it hard to resist that crusty French bread while waiting for a restaurant meal, ask the server not to bring the bread basket. Take the option out of the equation.

• Always ask for salad dressing on the side, and use it sparingly.

Learning to put on the brakes when you eat is an important step in adopting the Foundation lifestyle.

THE 90 PERCENT SOLUTION

Abiding by these guidelines for healthy eating will complement the Foundation work you are doing to make yourself flexible, strong, and pain free. For some of you, the changes in what you eat will be radical; for others, it will simply be a matter of tweaking, refining, and paying attention to what you already do. No matter what your eating habits are now, remember that no one is perfect. Take a clear-eyed look at your habits. The food log will help with that.

At the same time, you do not have to be completely rigid. There is no way you are going to turn down a piece of birthday cake at your child's party, a slice of pizza while watching a Monday night football game with friends, or a piece of your aunt's famous fried chicken. We are talking about eating clean, not being a food Nazi.

Some nutrition plans allow a "cheat day" every week. We do not recommend that approach, because you might just live to eat unhealthy things you crave that one day a week. You will still be dependent on food that is doing no good for your body. We prefer to apply the 90 percent rule. If you eat the way we suggest 90 percent of the time, you will be doing just fine. You will be giving your body more than enough nourishment to thrive.

After you have been eating clean for a month or so, the processed foods you used to crave will lose their appeal. They will no longer taste good to you, because you will have become accustomed to the subtle flavors and textures of simple, whole foods without additives, bad fats, corn syrup, and excessive salt.

CLEAN FOOD

The way you look is 70 to 80 percent based on what you eat. You can be fit, but the bottom line is that you will not look and feel great unless you eat well. Americans consume way too much processed, refined food. As food gets more processed, it becomes less like food. Our food is like astronaut food now, except space food distills nutrients and the food packaged in boxes and cans has had the natural nutrients wrung out and replaced with synthetic substitutes and corn syrup.

We cannot emphasize enough the importance of eating fresh vegetables and fruit, whole grains, and beef that has not been shot up with hormones. Since the pesticides and fertilizers used in commercial farming not only deplete the nutrients of plants but can also be harmful to your body, you should try to buy organic whenever possible. Though organically grown food can be more expensive, it is worth the additional cost to nourish your body with the most wholesome food that you can find.

We are not about to recommend a fad diet with no fat or no carbs. Health calls for balance—in nutrition and exercise. We advise you to eat what's known as a Paleolithic diet. You should eat what our ancient ancestors, the cave dwellers or hunter-gatherers, did: meat, fish, fresh vegetables, fruit, and nuts. Avoid processed, refined foods and just about any foods that are white. When you exercise strenuously, you need to eat carbohydrates to replenish your energy. Choose clean foods like yams, brown rice, and whole grains.

GOOD CARBS/BAD CARBS

When you eat carbs, your blood sugar rises—but just how much it does depends on the type of carbohydrate. Complex carbs like whole grains, most fruits and vegetables, and beans produce small, gradual increases. That's because they're rich in fiber, which slows digestion. When a food is digested slowly, energy is released gradually, supplying sustained energy with steady blood sugar levels. But refined or processed carbohydrates, like white rice or food made from white flour, cause rapid and big increases in blood sugar because the refining process removes much of the fiber. These easily digested foods cause blood sugar to spike. Your body produces insulin to drive down the blood sugar levels by stimulating cells to absorb the glucose, or sugar, in the bloodstream and store it as fat.

This dynamic, the rate at which a carbohydrate is broken down to glucose that enters the bloodstream, is measured by the glycemic index. The more quickly a food is digested, the higher its glycemic index. That's why you can eat a high-glycemic meal of pancakes and syrup and feel hungry an hour later. When a food takes longer to digest, the glycemic index will be lower and you will feel full longer.

Generally speaking, try to consume foods with a glycemic index below 40. A few examples will give you the picture.

Cornflakes 92	Croissant 67	Carrots 49
Scone 92	Oreo 64	Apple 38
Baked potato 85	Corn chips 63	Yams 37
Pretzels 83	Fresh corn 60	Broccoli 15
Gatorade 78	Cola 58	Asparagus 15
White rice 72	White pasta 50	Red peppers 10

Eating low–glycemic index carbohydrates will keep you full longer, give you a steady stream of energy, and help you avoid the peaks and valleys of fluctuating glucose levels that can cause you to crash during the day.

FOUNDATION'S ESSENTIAL CLEAN FOODS

Our approach to food is straightforward: Fresh, whole, and organic is the way to go. The list that follows offers an overview of the whole foods that provide your body with the nutrients it requires to function at the highest level.

Any and all vegetables: Really, do we have to tell you that you should be eating a lot of veggies? French fries don't count. Even though most of us have had this fact hammered into our brains, the only green food many folks eat is pickles. Organic vegetables are healthiest, and, generally, the less you cook them, the better. Eat them frequently. High-glycemic vegetables like corn, beets, and carrots should be eaten sparingly.

Greens: Our Paleolithic ancestors ate 6 pounds of leaves a day. Collard greens, chard, kale, mustard greens, and spinach are high in fiber, minerals, vitamins, and phytonutrients. Dark, leafy greens provide the most concentrated source of nutrients of any food. Greens just make you feel good.

Fruits: Though better for you than refined sugar, fruits can be high on the glycemic index and filled with natural sugar that is broken down quickly for energy. Make smart choices.

- **Berries** are great because they contain a lot of fiber and have powerful antioxidants.

- **Avocados** are excellent brain food, have 10 to 15 grams of fiber, and are high in healthy fats, lutein, vitamin K, folate, and a bunch of other good things. They also promote heart health.

- **Apples** contain many important nutrients. Among them: quercetin, a highly effective antioxidant that delays time to fatigue in elite athletes; creatine for muscles; fiber; and fructose. Eat an apple or two daily. Who cares about doctors? Do it for yourself.

• **Bananas** are high in fiber, vitamins B_6 and C, potassium, and manganese. They are high in sugar but help you feel full and give you energy. Potassium works to maintain fluid balance in the body. If you are working out hard and perspiring, potassium is a must.

Whole organic eggs: Go for the whole egg, because the yolk is packed with nutrients and healthy fats. If you are simply looking to get the protein, you are better off buying an albumin supplement of egg or hemp protein. Organic in this case will make a big difference. Buy cage free if you can.

Fresh fish: As a rule, the closer the fish was caught to its actual habitat, the better. Farm-raised fish does not follow a typical fishy diet or lifestyle and does not offer nearly as many of the healthy nutrients as wild fish, but it still has important nutrients. Get wild caught if you can, but if you can't, purchase fish that's as fresh as possible. It also helps to talk to the fish seller, who should be able to point you in the direction of the freshest fish.

Salmon gets its share of positive press, but there are many benefits to be had from other ocean and lake dwellers, too. Most types of fish have a decent amount of lean protein and healthy fats. The mercury and PCB content of shark, swordfish, king mackerel, tilefish, and tuna is high, so they should be avoided or eaten very infrequently. You should not eat more than two or three servings of fish a week.

Lean meat: We are meat eaters by nature, and meats—and by this we mean everything from red meat to chicken, turkey, pork, venison, and so on—do have a lot of muscle- and tissue-building proteins. The B vitamins they contain are important to our nervous systems. Though our lifestyles and functional demands have changed over the past handful of millennia, meat still has a central place on our menus. The difference is that it does not have to be the core component of our diet. We can sustain high energy with meat as an accessory or condiment—used sparingly.

Grains: Brown and wild rice are the starchy carbohydrates of choice. They have high fiber content and are digested slowly. Quinoa is another good option. This grain is an unusually complete protein source for a plant food. It has a 12 to 18 percent protein content due to its balanced set of amino acids.

Sprouted wheat bread: Better than whole wheat or white bread, sprouted wheat bread is digested more slowly and provides stable energy.

Yogurt: Stay away from the processed, sugar-filled kind and go for the good stuff. Greek and plain yogurts with live active cultures are what you're looking for. Generally, if the active cultures were added prior to the pasteurization process, they are dead and useless in terms of digestive assistance. When you check the ingredients list, make sure the bacteria were added after pasteurization. There are several reasonably priced varieties of healthful yogurts.

Seeds and nuts: To get the most out of almonds, cashews, pumpkin seeds, walnuts, and the rest, buy them raw. These are some of the healthiest snacks you can eat.

CLARITY ON THE GLUTEN-FREE TREND

We have noticed the term "gluten-free" lately in restaurants and on packaged foods everywhere. It's the new marketing buzzword in food. Sales for gluten-free products have risen exponentially in the past year. At this point, it is impossible to say if this is just another food trend that will pass as people focus on something else. Yet gluten intolerance is four times more common today than it was 50 years ago. No one knows exactly why, but some suspect that doctors are more aware of the condition now and thus are testing for it more than they used to.

Wheat, barley, rye, and oats contain the protein gluten. Some people have an autoimmune, inflammatory response in their small intestines when they eat grains containing gluten. In the case of gluten intolerance, undigested gluten proteins are treated like foreign invaders in the small intestine. The body turns on itself to expel the invaders, irritating the gut and damaging the villi, tiny projections on the lining of the small intestine. Consequently, there is less surface area in the small intestine to absorb nutrients from digested food.

The side effects of gluten intolerance are gastrointestinal distress, diarrhea, flatulence, bloating, constipation, headaches, joint pain, and fatigue. Celiac disease is an extreme form of gluten intolerance. The fallout from celiac disease can be serious, leading to chronic fatigue, serious nutritional deficiencies, anemia, nausea, rashes, and depression.

The good news is that the condition reverses once you stop eating gluten.

It is easy enough to test for gluten intolerance. Study your food log to see how much gluten you are consuming. If you have mild gastrointestinal symptoms regularly, try omitting wheat-, barley-, rye-, and oat-based flours. If your symptoms alleviate, you have an answer.

See your doctor if you have severe symptoms. There is a simple test to determine if you are intolerant to gluten.

ANTI-INFLAMMATORY FOODS

Inflammation is one of the key causes of pain. The Foundation lifestyle fights inflammation on all fronts, including nutrition. You will not find the foods that promote inflammation on our clean food list. Fast food, all varieties of junk food, sugar, high-fat meats, saturated and trans fats used in prepared and processed food, and nitrates all contribute to inflammation in your body.

Here is a quick reference to foods that are high in antioxidants and that combat inflammation.

Vegetables: arugula, asparagus, bean sprouts, bell peppers, bok choy, broccoli, broccoli rabe, Brussels sprouts, cabbage, cauliflower, chard, collards, cucumber, endive, escarole, garlic, green beans, kale, leeks, mushrooms, olives, onions, romaine lettuce, scallions, shallots, spinach, sweet potatoes, zucchini

Fruit: apples, avocados, blueberries, cantaloupe, cherries, clementines, guavas, honeydew melon, kiwifruit, kumquats, lemons, limes, oranges, papayas, peaches, pears, plums, raspberries, rhubarb, strawberries, tangerines, tomatoes

Animal proteins (preferably grass fed or wild): skinless and boneless chicken breast, turkey breast, anchovies, cod, halibut, herring, mackerel, oysters, rainbow trout, sablefish, salmon, sardines, shad, snapper, striped bass, tuna, whitefish

Nuts and seeds: almonds, flaxseed, hazelnuts, sunflower seeds, walnuts

Oils: extra-virgin olive oil, extra-virgin coconut oil

Herbs and spices: 70 percent cocoa, ginger, oregano, turmeric

Drinks: green tea, ginger tea, red wine (one glass a day)

EAT BREAKFAST LIKE A KING, LUNCH LIKE A PRINCE, AND DINNER LIKE A PAUPER

A "tapered diet" is the ideal way to eat; you should consume increasingly smaller meals throughout the day to allow your body and your digestive system to rest during your sleeping hours. We recommend eating six times a day: three meals and three snacks. Ideally, simple carbohydrates should be eaten only after strenuous workouts—and that means a minimum of 45 minutes at 65 to 95 percent effort that leaves you out of breath and tired—for optimal recovery. Right after a hard workout, you have a 30- to 60-minute window of increased absorption. Be honest with yourself. Including the right kinds of recovery-promoting carbs after serious workouts does not mean eating a bag of chips after a 40-minute stroll.

Your meals should include high protein and moderate amounts of healthy fat and complex carbohydrates. If you cannot resist simple carbohydrates, eat them only in the morning and after the tough workouts we mention above. Your carbohydrate intake should decline after 5:00 or 6:00 p.m., unless you are exercising hard after work. If you work out intensely late in the day, your body will need some carbohydrates to replenish energy stores.

We do not recommend low-fat diets. Essential fats actually help you lose weight. The right kind of fat is like WD-40 for your body. Healthy fats such as olive oil, avocado, almonds, and flaxseed should be part of your diet.

HOW TO BEGIN

Don't expect to change the way you eat overnight. You can't just boom, stop. This is not a fad diet that you stay on for a couple of weeks to lose a few pounds. We are talking about a major lifestyle change, and that does not happen cold turkey. Your body wants what it is used to. The process is like detox. It will take you a

YOUR DIET CAN HELP YOU GET A GOOD NIGHT'S SLEEP

You can raise the level of recovery and rejuvenation you get from sleep if you pay attention to what you eat in the evening. If your typical routine includes carbs, sugars, and a large meal before bed, there is a good chance you are inhibiting your brain's ability to secrete the proper amount of restful hormones.

Sugar is a stimulant, and infusing it into the digestive process triggers insulin and a host of other hormones that are used for going, not stopping. Most of our clients tell us that their food danger zone is after dinner, between 7:00 and 10:00 p.m. They may have eaten well all day, but then the night feeding begins. They can't resist a scoop of ice cream, some cookies, a bowl of cereal, or a piece of cake in the evening. By snacking on sweets and simple carbs, they are setting themselves up for sleep disturbance.

Aside from turning on your body when it should be relaxing, eating a big meal or unhealthy snack less than 3 hours before going to bed will contribute to weight problems. Those calories you have consumed will not be burned off and will be stored as you sleep.

Eat clean in the evening and you will sleep better at night.

month or so to adjust, because your body is going to crave that processed food. The first 2 weeks are the toughest. Once you start getting off junk food, you won't want it anymore. As soon as you break those habits, the thought of eating sweet, salty, greasy junk food will not even cross your mind.

Face it. You are going to be hungry at first. Learn to live with slight hunger. In fact, being a little bit hungry gives you an edge that can make you work better. Overeating can cause you to crash. You know that feeling after eating a big, heavy meal—all you can think about is a nap. Lean and hungry is a good thing.

To get started, look at your food log. Pick one thing that you'd like to change. Maybe instead of drinking four beers you elect to have one. You might break your cookie habit. We always suggest starting by cutting things. Pick one goal, achieve it, and move on to another. You might decide to eat at least one vegetable at each meal. Then you can commit to cutting out all white flours. It takes small steps, and then finally, over a period of 6 months or so, you are there.

It is difficult to control what you eat if you dine out a lot. Always ask that your food be prepared with as little oil as possible, pass on the bread, and have salad dressing on the side. Restaurants have become more accommodating as diners have become more health conscious.

Traveling can be even more of a challenge. We have seen people eating pizza in airports at 8:00 a.m. If you look hard enough, you can always find something healthy. If all else fails, go for almonds.

SNACKS ARE IMPORTANT

Snacks are crucial for maintaining energy throughout the day, but forget the cookies, crackers, and candy. To keep your energy up and feel satiated longer, eat snacks with a low glycemic index and with healthy fats. You should limit your snacks to about 300 calories. Consider a snack a holdover, not a mini-meal. These are some of the snacks we enjoy.

- A handful of almonds or other nuts with an apple or other fruit
- 2 ounces of sliced turkey or other lean meat
- A smoothie of 20 to 40 grams made with hemp, whey, chia seed, or egg protein and some frozen berries, with water as a base
- Veggies or beans with olive or sunflower oil dressing
- Hummus or another healthy bean dip on sprouted whole wheat or gluten-free toast or raw veggies

WATER: DRINK A LOT, DRINK FREQUENTLY, AND DRINK MORE

The more hydrated your body stays, the better it functions at every level, from the cells to the muscles to the organs. Many common daily ailments and low-energy issues can be partially remedied with better hydration. When you are dehydrated, your blood becomes viscous, which makes it difficult for all your organs and systems to perform normal tasks. Not drinking enough water puts a good deal of strain on your body.

Do your own experiment. Drink a full gallon of water each day for a week and see how you feel. The difference will be so noticeable that you will want to make a gallon a day a habit. Water will fill you up and make you less hungry. Sometimes what you perceive as hunger is actually thirst. If you feel hungry, have a glass of water. That might be all you need.

Natural juices not made from concentrates are fine, but the majority of fluid should be water. Caffeine and alcohol are dehydrating, so for every cup of coffee or drink you have, have a glass of water. For the most part, avoid energy drinks, sports drinks, and soda, because they are loaded with sugar and caffeine. Sports drinks

THE TEN RULES OF EATING

1. Eat to live, don't live to eat.

2. Log your food intake.

3. Eat a tapered diet—take smaller meals as the day goes on.

4. Practice portion control.

5. Eat only clean, nonprocessed food.

6. Eat a Paleolithic diet: lean meats, fish, vegetables, fruits, and nuts.

7. Determine your carbohydrate intake from your level of activity. After strenuous resistance training or high-intensity aerobic exercise lasting an hour or more, you must add some carbohydrate to facilitate recovery.

8. When changing your dietary habits, make adjustments in small steps. Each one will build upon the next, and before long you will make a concrete lifestyle change.

9. Hydrate properly. Drink 2 liters of water a day.

10. Follow these rules 80 percent of the time and you will be in great shape.

and gels can be used during and right after long-term aerobic exercise of an hour or more.

A DAY'S MEAL PLAN

We want to give you an idea of what clean eating looks like for a day. There is such a great variety of food you can enjoy that you should consider these meals only a suggestion of the way to eat.

BREAKFAST

Have this meal soon after you wake up to get your metabolism on the upstroke. The meal should consist of complex carbs, healthy fat, and good protein. Try to make vegetables a part of your breakfast. Since most of us have breakfast on the run, here are a few easy-to-prepare meals that will start your day the right way.

- Banana or apple with 1 to 2 tablespoons of sunflower or almond butter

- Egg and vegetable omelet (perhaps using leftover veggies from dinner) with fresh berries. If trying to cut calories, use one egg and three egg whites. If exercising strenuously, add a piece of sprouted wheat or brown rice bread.

- Smoothie with almond milk, frozen berries, high-quality protein powder, and some flaxseed, chia seed, or almond butter

- Oatmeal with high-quality protein powder and a tablespoon of peanut butter (a good choice on the days you exercise strenuously)

MIDMORNING SNACK

You want to sustain your energy throughout the morning. A healthy snack will keep your energy high and prevent you from being ravenous at lunchtime. Try to keep snacks under 300 calories.

- A handful of almonds or other nuts and some fruit

- 2 ounces of turkey or other lean meat and a small piece of fruit

- Apple and a tablespoon or two of sunflower, almond, or peanut butter

LUNCH

Do your best to stay away from simple carbs at midday. They will make you feel sluggish after lunch. The more water you drink at this time of day, the better you will feel in general.

- Organic chicken breast or fish seasoned with olive oil and herbs and ½ avocado or other veggies

- Large mixed green salad made with lean meat, veggies, and avocado (no cheese). Use dressing sparingly, and avoid heavy types.

- Half of a turkey and avocado sandwich with small mixed green salad

- Fresh chicken and vegetable soup

AFTERNOON SNACK

Most people are low in energy at midafternoon. Having a nutritious snack will pick you up.

- A handful of raw nuts with an apple or other fruit

- Raw veggies and hummus

- Raw, organic energy bar

DINNER

If you want to sleep well, stay away from rice and pasta at this meal. Avoid starchy carbs.

- Grass-fed beefsteak and a salad

- A large stir-fry or vegetable-based dinner with shrimp, chicken, or tofu added

- Roast chicken with asparagus, green beans, or broccoli and a green salad

- Grilled wild salmon with veggies and a green salad

BEFORE BED

- A square of dark chocolate (70 percent cocoa) if you have a craving for sweets

- A handful of nuts

- A cup of herbal tea

- Unsweetened almond or hemp milk with a teaspoon of chia seeds

DRINK OPTIONS

- Minimum of 2 liters of water a day

- Fresh-pressed juices

- A cup or two of coffee

- As much herbal tea as you want. Limit your intake of green, black, or white tea—they contain caffeine.

- Almond, hemp, rice, or oat milk—stay away from dairy varieties of milk

- Avoid diet sodas. Artificial sweeteners are addictive and make you crave sweetness. They also set off an insulin response in your body, which makes you store the energy you consume as fat. If you must use a sweetener, we recommend stevia, an all-natural herbal sweetener.

Putting Foundation principles of clean eating in your life will give you the energy and the stamina to go beyond Foundation workouts and build a varied exercise plan that will bring you to a higher level of fitness.

10

TRAINING THE
FOUNDATION WAY

MAKING YOUR WORKOUT WORK FOR YOU

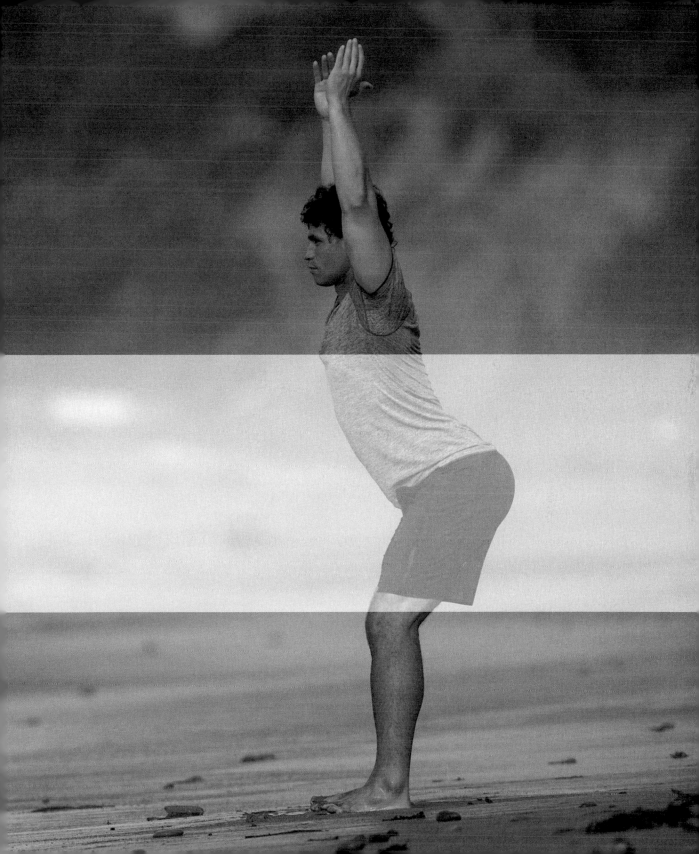

Once you have completed the 6-week Foundation program, you will not believe how great you feel. You'll be moving the way your body is meant to. Your body will be primed to do more. Foundation exercises are the base of your training, and now it is time to build on the workouts and see how far you can go. You can take Foundation training to any exercise, sport, or traditional weight program. Doing basic movements correctly will make you more powerful, agile, and flexible. You'll find traditional exercise programs and everything you do much easier.

> You can take Foundation training to any exercise, sport, or traditional weight program. Doing basic movements correctly will make you more powerful, agile, and flexible.

Inactivity might have been the root cause of your back pain. Don't revert to being sedentary once your back pain goes away. Foundation exercises should become a part of your life and routine. If you don't keep up with the training, there is a good chance your back will act up again. You have to keep your back and posterior chain powerful to prevent flare-ups. Seeing what Foundation training has done for your body in only 6 weeks should motivate you to make exercise and fitness an important part of your life. You deserve the benefits that regular exercise will deliver.

THE BENEFITS OF EXERCISE

We know you've heard it all before, but we want to highlight why regular exercise is so important and all the good things physical activity does for you. Exercise will help you to:

- Boost metabolism.
- Lose weight and keep it off.
- Look and feel younger.
- Sleep better.
- Reduce stress and muscle tension.
- Build and maintain healthy bones, muscles, and joints.
- Release negative emotions like anger and hostility.
- Alleviate depression and anxiety by raising endorphin levels that produce a "runner's high."
- Lower your risk of developing heart disease, diabetes, high blood pressure, and cancer.
- Reverse or improve those serious conditions.
- Raise self-esteem.
- Increase body awareness.

Regular exercise is one of the most important things you can do for yourself. Since you already have issues with your muscles, bones, and joints, exercise is even more essential in your life. You can lose weight and look good and still feel bad. If you have weight to lose, that is just the beginning. Your emphasis should be on changing your movement and then moving more; all of the other good things will come from there.

If you already exercise regularly, you know how easy it is to get hooked. For those of you who do not need to be persuaded, we will share some tips to help you boost your metabolism and make your exercise more efficient.

If you haven't been exercising, ask yourself a simple question: *Why don't I exercise?* Consider what obstacles slow you down. Do you hate the gym? Are you self-conscious there because you are out of shape? Are you afraid of reinjuring yourself?

You've got options. No one says you have to go to a gym. You could take a walk, ride a bike, jump rope, go dancing, play tennis, swim laps, get a yoga tape and practice at home; the possibilities are endless. If you do something you enjoy, it will be easier to start.

The excuse we hear most often is "I just don't have the time." Why not schedule slots of time to do the activity of your choice? Many people work one-on-one with a trainer because they have made an appointment and it is on their calendar. Having an exercise buddy can also be a great help. It's harder to blow off a workout if someone is expecting you. A little quiet competition never hurts, either.

There is almost always a way to carve out time to exercise. Do you spend your leisure time sitting in front of the tube? Get some free weights and work out while you watch. Can you wake up earlier and get outside to walk, run, or bike? Starting your morning with exercise sets you up for the entire day. Can you leave your desk at lunch to take a walk? How about reserving some time before dinner? You could take a yoga class to unwind or do aerobics at the gym. Exercise does not have to be torturous. What is important is to do something that works for you. After a few weeks, you will feel like a different person. You'll forget how sluggish you were before you changed your life.

You have to make exercise part of your routine. It doesn't take long to form a habit, especially when it has such positive results. Some of our clients like to exercise at the same time every day, at least when they start working out, to reinforce the habit. First thing in the morning seems to work best for most people. That's because it's easy to get caught up in other things as the day goes on, so if you are

FOUNDATIONFIRST
THE FOUNDATION WAY OF LIFE

Peter Park's holistic approach evolves his training into a way of life. His background as a professional athlete and his passion for exercise, sports, and fitness have given him an in-depth knowledge of the human body and make him a particularly gifted trainer. It is no surprise that on his roster, Peter has some of the best athletes on the planet and in such diverse fields as cycling, surfing, and basketball. Peter's approach to training is unique—he understands your issues, goals, and motivations and will challenge you to bring out your best to reach them.

I met Peter after a terrible car accident, when I thought that I would not be able to practice the sports I used to or simply enjoy my old way of life. Physical therapy got me stable but nowhere near healthy. Working with Peter, combined with learning Foundation exercises, has taken my body as far as it is capable of going. I am back to surfing, hiking, and other activities that make life good. Thanks to Peter, the impossible became possible, and in a way he has given my life back to me.

OLAF GUERRAND-HERMES

absorbed by work and other worries, you might be too distracted to focus on your body as you exercise. To have a good workout, you have to pay attention to what you are doing. You can always get up earlier to squeeze a workout into a busy schedule. You will also be freshest right after you wake up. Plus, if you exercise early in the morning, you will rev up your metabolism and mood for hours after. You couldn't ask for a better way to start the day.

If you are not a morning person and dread the thought of dragging yourself out of bed to exercise, you can at least make sure you take a lunch break and go for a walk. Get up from that desk and get moving. You could use the time immediately following work to exercise and unwind. Exercising before dinner can be a great transition from work to home. Whatever time of day you work out, once you get into it, it will start to seem less like a chore and become something you look forward to every day; once you get into it, you'll discover that working out is a reward loop that is hard to resist.

Whether you are just beginning, starting up again, or continuing your commitment to work out regularly, it is a good idea to work with a trainer for a session or two to develop a workout plan that will suit your needs and keep you challenged. A professional trainer will be able to evaluate your level of fitness and flexibility and tailor a program that will produce maximum results. Consulting with a trainer will take the guesswork out of the process.

Don't just go to any gym and work with whoever is around. Ask friends, acquaintances, even your doctor for a referral. Word of mouth is the best way to find a good trainer.

THE PERFECT WEEK

In addition to your three or four Foundation workouts a week, you should do resistance training twice a week and cardio at least three times a week. We tell our clients to do a long aerobic workout for an hour or more, 1 day a week, preferably outside. During the weekend, walk, jog, run, hike, go in-line skating, or ride a bike for an hour or more. Do anything that is continuous. Don't sit on an exercise bike reading a magazine: Get out in the fresh air. Build to 1½ or 2 hours. Move at a comfortable pace. The goal is to build your endurance.

Here are a few additional guidelines for a balanced program.

• You should do nothing 1 or 2 days a week. Your body needs the recovery time. Since most of our clients find it easier to work out on the weekend, we chose Wednesday as the recovery day for our perfect week. The obligations and demands in your life will shape your week.

• You can do your workouts all at once each day or break them up, depending on the time available to you.

• Your two resistance-training sessions should be separated by 48 hours. When you train with weights, microtears occur in your muscles. Spacing out your resistance training will allow your muscles to repair and rebuild.

• Take a recovery week every 4th or 5th week by reducing your intensity by 40 to 50 percent. Give your body and mind a break. More about overtraining later.

Do not be a slave to your schedule. If you do not feel good after 10 minutes of working out, shut it down. Learn to manage your fatigue. If you are not feeling good after working out, you are not progressing. You need to evaluate what you are doing. Are you working out with too much intensity? Are you scheduling insufficient recovery time? Your intention is not to punish your body. That will break it down. The Foundation lifestyle is all about balance and not pushing too hard. Pushing too hard might well be the reason you had back pain to begin with.

The schedule that follows is a suggestion of how a week should look. What is good for one person is not necessarily right for another. You have to make exercise an integral part of your life. Develop a flexible schedule that takes into account the demands of your life and your energy levels throughout the day. There are always reasons to postpone a workout. You have to commit to a reasonable level of exercise to stay healthy and feel good.

SUNDAY	MONDAY	TUESDAY	WEDNESDAY	THURSDAY	FRIDAY	SATURDAY
Foundation 20–30 min or day off	Cardio interval 20 min	Foundation 20–30 min	Recovery day	Foundation 20–30 min	Foundation 20–30 min	Long cardio 1–3 hr
	Resistance 30 min			Resistance 30 min	Cardio interval 20 min	

WITHOUT RECOVERY, THERE IS NO PROGRESS

Just as you eased into changing your eating habits, you should take it slow when you begin to exercise and build gradually. We have seen so many people start with the pedal to the metal. They are gung ho and push hard every day at the beginning of an exercise program. They can handle it for about 2 months. Sooner or later, they come to the gym, and they look wasted. Then they never come back. They overtrain and burn out.

When you overtrain, you are not allowing enough recovery time. Recovery enables your body to regenerate. If you do a really hard workout and go hard again the next day and the next, your body will be in a constant state of breakdown. We recommend 48 hours between hard workouts. Your muscles need time to rest and regenerate.

HOW ELITE ATHLETES RECOVER AND REGENERATE

Aside from using food to restore their bodies, athletes utilize a number of techniques to speed their recovery from strenuous physical effort. You can do the same for yourself.

To ease muscle pain and relax your muscles, try the proven methods of the list that follows:

1. For a quick recovery, take a cold plunge. Some athletes dump bags of ice into their cold baths.

2. Ice the area of your body that is affected, especially an aching back.

3. Use a foam roller for self-massage (instructions at the end of this chapter).

4. Have a professional do tissue work.

5. Get a lot of sleep.

6. Walk at a relaxed pace to loosen up.

Remember, you will not improve unless you allow yourself to recover.

Overtraining is wasted training. We tell our clients that it is better to be

> Overtraining is almost as bad as not training at all.

a little undertrained than it is to be over-trained. If you over-train, you are going to crave sugar. You will get depressed, lethargic, and moody. Your heart rate will stay elevated, and you won't sleep well. Overtraining is almost as bad as not training at all.

STOP MUSCLE LOSS

Our ancestors had to push their muscles hard in order to survive. From the hunter-gatherers to the farmers of the agrarian age to the housewives and manual laborers of the early 20th century, they had to expend a tremendous amount of physical effort in everyday life. Getting from one place to another took a lot of energy. Today we take for granted the automation and conveniences that make industry and everyday chores less demanding. As a result of all of the technological advances, we have to make a conscious choice to work our muscles.

Unless they do something about it, most people lose 5 pounds of muscle and gain 10 pounds of fat for every decade after age 30. One of the ways to protect and build muscle mass is resistance training. Resistance training—or strength training, as it is also called—causes muscles to contract against an external force. That could mean weights, exercise bands, or your own body weight. The contraction against resistance creates microtears in your muscle tissue, a catabolic breakdown of muscle. When allowed recovery time, those tiny tears are repaired and your muscles grow, a process known as anabolism. Aside from building muscles, resistance training builds bone (which also declines with age), helps lower high blood pres-

FOUNDATIONFIRST

I am fortunate enough to represent some of the world's greatest athletes, and after working with Peter and Eric for the last 2 years, I am starting to feel as strong as one! The core principles of this book have made me stronger and fitter than I ever imagined possible, and I intend to make them a part of my daily routine for many years to come.

CASEY WASSERMAN, CHAIRMAN AND CEO OF WASSERMAN MEDIA GROUP

sure, and raises metabolism. Well-toned and healthy muscles will enable you to move well and will brace your back and joints, preventing painful imbalances.

MAKE A LIGHT WEIGHT SEEM HEAVY: TIPS ON RESISTANCE TRAINING

The best strength-training programs employ full-body compound movements, multijoint exercises, and hip hinging. Moves like squats, deadlifts, pushups, and pullups give you more bang for your buck because multiple muscle groups are used simultaneously. Not only is this training more functional, but working in this manner is metabolically demanding and will burn more calories.

Stay away from isolation exercises such as biceps curls, triceps extensions, and leg curls, which work one small area and have a very small metabolic demand. If you are new to weight training, learn to master the Foundation movements and bodyweight exercises such as pullups, pushups, squats, and the hip hinge before adding resistance. Once you are comfortable with the basics, following a few simple rules will keep your resistance training safe and efficient.

• Strength training is a skill. Focus on proper technique at all times.

• Vary the number of sets and repetitions that you do. The fewer the reps, the more sets are necessary. You generally want to aim for 15 to 20 reps per exercise. For example, one day you may do 4 sets of 5 reps and another day 2 sets of 10 reps. The rep range will determine your goals. If you are looking for strength, stay primarily in the 3- to 8-rep range; if you are looking to gain some hypertrophy or size, stay in the 10- to 15-rep range; and for strength endurance, you can go up to 20 to 25 reps.

• Don't be afraid of doing lower reps and using heavier weights. Women especially tend to shy away from heavier weights for fear of bulking up, but doing a lower number of reps will actually build muscle strength, not mass. Lift the heaviest weight you can manage with complete control and perfect technique. Stop 1 to 2 reps before muscle failure and you will recover faster, progress further, and reduce your chance of injury.

• The way you perform an exercise is just as important as which exercise you choose to do. Aim for great technique with perfect movement when doing your resistance training. Always take the movement through the full range of motion and lock out the joints in order to strengthen them the same way you strengthen muscles.

• Keeping tension in the body while lifting can help your strength by up to 20 percent. When you are lifting a weight, keep your breath very shallow and allow tension in your entire body. It doesn't matter how light the weight is. Strive to make even the lightest weight feel heavy by creating tension. If you compare an Olympic weight lifter to a beginner, you'll see what we mean. The Olympic lifter will have full-body tension and complete control, while the beginner will look loose and vulnerable. It's extremely important to focus on this during your strength sessions. Lifting in this fashion will keep your muscles tight, decrease power leaks, and stabilize the movement you are performing. When you lose tension while lifting, you become weaker and more susceptible to injury.

• To make your workouts productive and efficient, you should train in circuits of opposing muscle groups. For example, a typical workout may look like this—circuit 1: 5 sets of 5 reps of shoulder press and pullups; circuit 2: 5 sets of 5 reps of squats and deadlifts; circuit 3: 5 sets of 5 reps of shoulder press and rows.

Resistance training just twice a week will build your muscles and prevent the muscle loss that comes with aging.

THE MOST EFFICIENT WAY TO TRAIN

You do not have to spend hours on a treadmill or elliptical machine dreading every minute, counting the seconds until you are finished. Short duration, high-intensity

CALCULATING YOUR TRAINING ZONES

We prefer the Karvonen method of calculating your target heart rate for various training zones, because it is much more accurate than, for example, the common formula of simply using your maximum heart rate by subtracting your age from 220 and then calculating your training zones from that number. The common formula does not take your resting heart rate into account.

This is how to get a more accurate guideline of how hard you have to work to get the most from exercise.

Step 1: Find Your Resting Heart Rate

Take your pulse 15 minutes after you wake up in the morning and before you get out of bed. Count your pulse for 10 seconds and multiply by six. That number is your resting heart rate. You can find your pulse by putting two fingers on the thumb side of your wrist or below your jaw along the windpipe in your neck.

Do this three mornings in a row. Add those numbers together, and divide the sum by three to get your average resting heart rate. For example:

76 + 72 + 74 = 222 ÷ 3 = 74 average resting heart rate

Make sure to take your pulse after a recovery day. The results will be affected if you try to find your resting heart rate after strenuously working out the day before.

Step 2: Find Your Maximum Heart Rate

Subtract your age from 220 to find your maximum heart rate. Let's say you are 30 years old:

training is both more stimulating and effective than the typical routine of 30 to 60 minutes at a moderate pace. With interval training, you alternate bursts of intense activity with periods of easy recovery. As with strength training, you have

220 − 30 = 190 = maximum heart rate

Step 3: Find Your Heart Rate Reserve

Subtract your average resting heart rate from your maximum heart rate. For example:

190 − 74 = 116 = heart rate reserve

Step 4: Calculate Your Training Zones

The target heart rate for a standard cardio workout is somewhere between 60 and 80 percent. If you want to calculate the lower limit for your cardio target heart rate, multiply your heart rate reserve number by 0.6, and add your resting heart rate to the answer. If you want the upper limit for your cardio target heart rate, multiply the number you reached in step 3 by 0.8, and add your resting heart rate to the answer. For example:

116 × 0.6 + 74 = 143.6 = low end of your cardio target rate
116 × 0.8 + 74 = 166.2 = high end of your cardio target rate

When you do interval training, you will aim for a higher heart rate because you will be exerting yourself more.

116 × 0.9 + 74 = 178.4 = target heart rate for 90 percent exertion

to vary the workout. You can switch between longer intervals of 3 to 10 minutes at 80 to 85 percent effort and shorter, more powerful intervals of 15 seconds to 1 minute at up to 95 percent effort. A typical interval workout would be 20 to 30 minutes in length. You will build a stronger, more powerful cardiovascular system with interval training.

When you work at high intensity, the exercise is anaerobic, or without oxygen. Your body uses glycogen stored in your muscles for fuel. Lactic acid is a byproduct of this process. At the same time, you build an oxygen debt. During the recovery periods your body is trying to recover by flushing lactic acid out of the muscles. Interval training speeds up this process by promoting the building of new capillaries to get oxygen to and waste products from the muscles. The more oxygen you can get to your muscles and the faster you can flush out lactate, the more aerobically fit you will become.

High-intensity training integrated into a typical workout routine will yield a significantly higher afterburn, the increase in metabolic rate after exercising. Your body will keep that heightened state of efficiency for several hours after a 20-minute workout, and you will burn more calories with your everyday activity. Interval training will turn your body into a fuel-burning machine. Another benefit is that your high heart rate will produce endorphins, which will make you feel good for the rest of the day.

Our advice is to stay out of what we call junk pace, which is the middle ground. It is much more efficient to alternate between hard and easy. Keeping a monotonous middle pace can be counterproductive. A junk pace will not raise your heart rate very high, but it still requires recovery. Since you have not pushed hard, you might not feel you need recovery time. You can end up overtraining and burning out. If you run at the same pace for an extended period day after day, your body adjusts to the demand, and you burn fewer calories as a consequence. Interval training makes so much more sense.

Some people—you know the type—are not able to go easy. Driven, intense people have no problem training full out. If they could learn to take it slow for recovery, they would be amazed by what they could achieve.

WORKOUTS FOR BECOMING A FUEL-BURNING MACHINE

You can do interval training anywhere. You go from easy effort to bursts of intense effort, from walking to jogging or jogging to running, depending on your level of fitness. You can take it outside by finding a hill near where you live. Walk up as fast as you can, and then walk down at a slower pace. If you do that for 20 minutes, you will get a great workout. If you are working out on a treadmill or elliptical machine, you can do 2 minutes easy and 30 seconds hard and repeat those intervals. Just play with the intervals. Interval training will save you time and produce significantly higher benefits for the time you invest. If you want to take the guesswork out of it, you should invest in a heart rate monitor, which will let you know if you are working out in your target training zones.

Here are a number of cardio interval workouts for you to try.

FIVE INTERVAL WORKOUTS FOR THE ELLIPTICAL

When most people use an elliptical machine, they power the movement from their toes, their quads doing most of the work. Using Foundation principles, place your weight on your heels while holding an upright posture, so that your hamstrings and glutes are propelling the movement. Avoid leaning on the machine by maintaining a light grip.

WARMUP

1. For each of the elliptical workouts, begin with 3 to 5 minutes of easy, low resistance with high strides per minute, which is called faster stride turnover.

2. Do 3 × 30-second controlled sprints, followed by a 30-second recovery. Make each sprint a bit faster.

3. Take 1 to 2 minutes easy before beginning intervals.

WORKOUT 1

1. 4 × 1 minute at 80 to 85 percent effort with a 1-minute recovery. Keep resistance at medium difficulty and strides per minute high.

2. 4 × 30 seconds at 85 to 90 percent effort with a 1-minute recovery. Set resistance a bit higher; try to keep strides up.

3. 4 × 15 seconds at 90 to 95 percent effort with a 45-second recovery. Increase resistance a bit more, and push these hard.

WORKOUT 2: **IN AND OUTS**

1. Do a 2-minute interval, with 1 minute at high resistance and ramp (if machine has ramp), then 1 minute at lower resistance and fast strides.

2. Take a 1-minute recovery.

3. Do five more intervals.

WORKOUT 3: **INCREASING STRIDES**

1. Start with a medium to easy effort level of resistance and stride speed.

2. Every minute, bring the resistance level up by one level while trying to hold the same strides per minute.

3. Continue to increase resistance until you are unable to hold strides per minute. If you went longer than 5 minutes, you started too easy; less than 3 minutes, you started too hard.

4. Aim for 4 to 5 minutes per interval. Take 1 to 2 minutes recovery and continue the pattern for 12 to 20 minutes.

WORKOUT 4: **TIME TRIAL**

Go 15 minutes at 80 to 90 percent effort. Mark your distance and note how much farther you get as you get fitter.

WORKOUT 5: **MIXED-PACE INTERVALS**

1. Do a 4-minute steady tempo interval at 80 to 85 percent effort.

2. Take a 1-minute rest.

3. Do 4 × 15 seconds at 95 percent effort with a 45-second recovery.

4. Do two rounds.

FIVE INTERVAL WORKOUTS FOR THE BIKE

Doing your cardio work on a stationary bike is not optimal for most people because cycling reinforces the rounded shoulder-forward head posture that Foundation training is trying to address. Interval training on the bike is great—just make sure to mix it up with other forms of cardio. Do not spend hours in the gym on the exercise bike reinforcing bad movement and posture problems.

If you do use a stationary bike, make sure you keep your spine extended. Sit tall and hinge from your hips. Make sure the seat is at the proper height. To check, sit on the bike with your heels on the pedals, then pedal backward. At the bottom of the revolution, your knees should be slightly bent. You should be able to keep your hips still when you pedal. Press the pedals with your heels rather than your toes to activate your posterior chain.

WARMUP

1. For each of the cycling workouts, begin with 5 minutes of easy, low resistance with high cadence.

2. Do 3 or 4 × 30 second controlled sprints using moderate resistance while maintaining a high cadence (90 to 110 rpm).

3. Take 1 to 2 minutes easy before starting your intervals.

WORKOUT 1: **FLAT/HILL INTERVALS**

1. Do 8 × 1 minute hard with a 1-minute recovery.

2. Do even intervals (flat) with medium resistance and high rpm (90+), and odd intervals (hills) with high resistance and lower rpm.

WORKOUT 2: **VARIED-PACE INTERVALS**

1. Do 16 minutes with 1 minute at a "comfortably hard" pace alternating with 1 minute at a challenging pace.

2. The key is to transition from pace to pace without having to rest.

WORKOUT 3: **HALF-MILE REPEATS**

1. Do ½ mile at 80 to 90 percent with a 1-minute rest.

2. Try to make each interval faster than the previous, so do not start too fast!

3. Do as many repeats as you can in 16 to 20 minutes.

WORKOUT 4: **DROP-SET INTERVALS**

During this 20-minute workout, intervals should be more intense as the interval gets shorter.

1. 5 minutes hard, 2 minute recovery

2. 4 minutes hard, 2 minute recovery

3. 3 minutes hard, 1 minute recovery

4. 2 minutes hard, 1 minute recovery

5. 1 minute hard, 1 minute off

WORKOUT 5: **TIME TRIAL**

Go 15 minutes at 90 to 95 percent effort. Mark your distance and see how much farther you go as you get fitter.

FIVE INTERVAL WORKOUTS FOR THE TREADMILL

Depending on your level of fitness, you can walk, jog, or run as you do these treadmill workouts.

WARMUP

1. For each of the treadmill workouts, begin with 5 minutes of easy running.

2. Do 3 to 4 pickups of 30 seconds to prepare for the upcoming harder efforts. Make each pickup a bit faster.

3. Take 1 to 2 minutes easy before beginning intervals.

WORKOUT 1: **HILL REPEATS**

1. Do 5 × 1 minute at an incline of 6 to 7 percent at 80 to 85 percent effort with a 1-minute recovery.

2. Do 5 × 30 seconds at an incline of 6 to 7 percent at 85 to 90 percent effort with a 1-minute recovery.

WORKOUT 2: **DESCENDING INTERVALS**

The goal is to go a bit faster as the interval gets shorter. Try to make it one continuous set, taking 1-minute rests.

1. 2 × 1½ minutes at 80 to 85 percent effort with a 1-minute recovery

2. 2 × 1¼ minutes at 80 to 85 percent with a 1-minute recovery

3. 2 × 1 minute at 85 to 90 percent with a 1-minute recovery

4. 2 × 45 seconds at 85 to 90 percent with a 1-minute recovery

5. 2 × 30 seconds at 85 to 90 percent with a 1-minute recovery

WORKOUT 3: **PACE-CHANGE INTERVALS**

1. Do 3 minutes at 75 to 80 percent effort.

2. Do 3 × 30 seconds at 90 to 95 percent effort with 1-minute break in between.

3. Recover for 1½ to 2 minutes.

4. Repeat for a total of three rounds.

WORKOUT 4: **HILL/FLAT INTERVALS**

1. Do a 1-minute hill interval at a 5 to 7 percent incline at 80 to 85 percent effort.

2. Go right into 1 minute flat at 80 to 85 percent effort.

3. Recover for 1 to 1½ minutes and repeat for six to eight intervals.

WORKOUT 5: **RUN TIME TRIAL**

Run or walk at 80 to 85 percent effort for 15 minutes. See how much farther you run as you get fitter.

FIVE ROWING INTERVAL WORKOUTS

We love the rowing machine, because the movement is the opposite of the position most of us are in all day. Rowing promotes good posture and reinforces Foundation principles. When you are rowing, it is important to keep tall in your spine and hinge from your hips. Most people do not realize that 70 percent of rowing should come from the legs. At the bottom of the stroke, you push out with your legs and your arms follow. The movement from the top of the stroke is recovery. During this phase your body relaxes as you let your arms out first, and then follow with bending legs. For great visuals of technique and workout ideas, go to www.concept2.com.

WARMUP

1. For each of the rowing workouts, begin with 3 to 5 minutes of easy rowing, working on perfect technique.

2. Do a few 20- to 30-second sprints to elevate your heart rate and prepare for more intense work.

3. Take 1 to 2 minutes easy before beginning intervals.

WORKOUT 1: **DESCENDING INTERVALS**

The pace should quicken as intervals get shorter.

1. 1 × 1,000 meters at 80 to 85 percent effort, 1 minute rest

2. 2 × 500 meters at 80 to 85 percent effort, 1 minute rest

3. 3 × 250 meters at 80 to 85 percent effort, 1 minute rest

WORKOUT 2: **POWER SET**

1. 4 × 250 meters at 85 to 90 percent effort

2. 5 × 100 meters at 90 to 95 percent effort, 1 minute rest

WORKOUT 3: **PACE INTERVALS**

Do 3 to 5 × 1,000 meters at 85 percent effort with a 1½-minute rest. Keep your stroke long and work on perfect technique.

WORKOUT 4: **THRESHOLD SET**

Do 6 to 10 × 250 meters at 80 to 85 percent effort with a 30-second recovery. Try to maintain a hard pace for all intervals.

WORKOUT 5: **ROWING TIME TRIAL**

Row a 2,000-meter time trial at 80 to 85 percent effort, and note the distance so you can see improvement as your fitness progresses.

THE BEST WORKOUT FOR YOU IS ONE YOU HAVE NEVER DONE

Your body is a remarkable machine designed to preserve itself and conserve energy. If you do the same workout repeatedly, your body will adapt to the demand, and your metabolism will not rise as high as it used to. The result is that the same effort will burn fewer calories. Peter has run so many miles in his career that he probably burns half the calories of someone who is just beginning to jog. The same adjustment happens when you diet. If you reduce your caloric intake, your body goes into starvation mode. Your metabolism slows down to get the most from the available calories. Our message is that you have to change it up. You have to row one day, do a spin class, run, walk on the treadmill, learn to box, jump rope, throw a medicine ball around, try something new. Don't go to the gym and use the same machines for the same length of time at the same pace. The idea with cardio training is to work your body in ways it does not expect. Confusing your body will keep your metabolism buzzing.

CHANGE IT UP

Getting stuck in a rut with your exercise program is the last thing you want to do. You want your exercise to count, and the way to ensure that your efforts are paying off big is to vary your workouts. Have fun with it. There is so much you can do to get your heart rate up and your metabolism pumped. Here are just a few ideas.

Aerobic dance	Jumping rope	Swimming
Basketball	Kickboxing	Tennis
Biking	Rowing machine	Treadmill
Circuit classes	Soccer	VersaClimber
Cross-country skiing	Spinning	Walking
Elliptical machine	Squash	Water aerobics
In-line skating	Stepmill	Yoga
Jogging	Surfing	

A routine can become comfortable, and that is not what you want. Varying your exercise will keep you from getting bored, shake up the status quo, and raise your metabolic baseline.

FOAM ROLLING: THE POOR MAN'S MASSAGE

Professional athletes need a team of physical therapists, massage therapists, and chiropractors to work their muscles to relieve muscle tension and aches and pains. There is a simple way for you to get the knots out of your muscles that does not require the services of a pro. Foam rolling can do the job. A foam roll is a dense foam cylinder, 6 inches in diameter and 36, 18, or 12 inches long, that resembles a pool noodle. By applying your body weight to the foam roller in specific spots, you can give your soft tissue a massage and relieve tight muscles. The tender spots in your muscles are called knots, or trigger points. If you use the foam roller to massage these knots, you will increase bloodflow to your tissue, which becomes suppler and moves better.

We are reminded of a 100-meter sprinter who had a chronic problem with hamstring pulls. We had watched the way he trained. He was in such great shape that he could put his elbows on the ground when stretching his hamstrings. That means his injury was not a length issue but a tissue problem. He probably had developed knots in the belly of his hamstrings. When his hamstrings contracted during his sprint, the muscle pulled on either side of a knot, and he was injured. A foam roller workout would have loosened the tissue and might have prevented that pull.

We expect all of our clients to do 5 to 10 minutes of foam rolling before they work out. Self-massage will prepare your muscles to work hard. You can even do it when you watch TV at night. Getting rid of those knots might help you get a better night's sleep.

A foam roller can cost less than $25. We prefer the Trigger Point foam roller, which is only 13 inches long. It is a bit more expensive than most foam rollers, but it is durable and well designed. Trigger Point Performance Therapy offers a number of high-end rollers that look like barbells for specific areas. If you have chronic

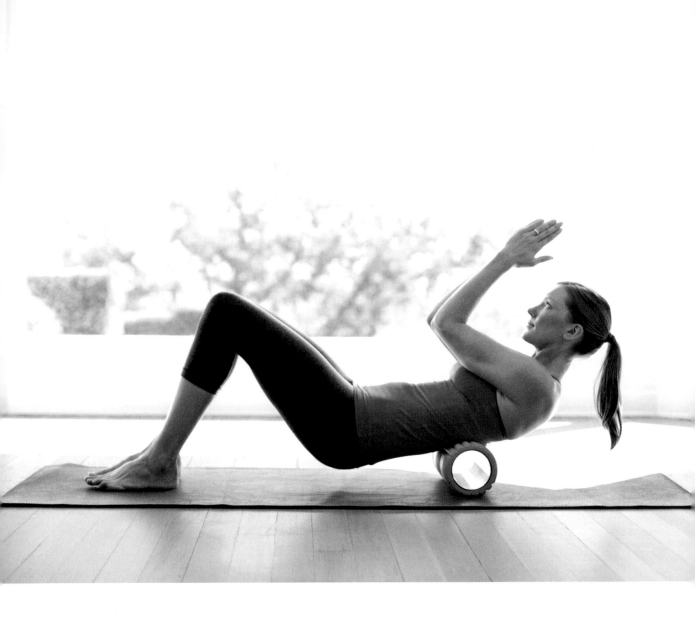

lower-back pain, you might want to invest in one designed for that area of the body.

Short foam rollers are also great to pack and take with you when you travel. Sitting for hours in the tight space of a plane seat can make you very stiff. If you are working a small area like your calves, you can use a tennis or lacrosse ball.

FOAM ROLLER WORKOUT

You might feel awkward when you first try these exercises, but it should not take you long to master the foam roller. You know the places where you feel knots in your muscles: calves, hamstrings, adductors, IT band, glutes, quads, hip flexors, lats, pecs, upper spine, and lower back. These exercises will show you how to get to those knots. Many clients say this is their favorite part of a workout. It is a great way to develop body awareness and prepare you for a good work session. You can adjust the pressure by how much you support your weight with your arms. Do triage with your foam roller wherever you are tight.

CALVES

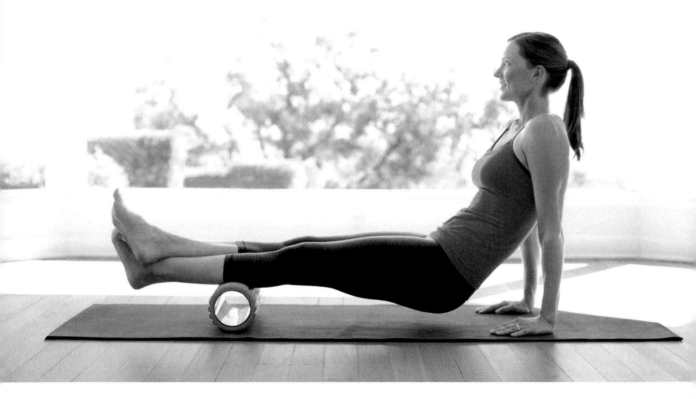

① Sit with the roller under your left calf with your right leg bent. Lean back with straight arms, supporting your weight with your hands. Flex your left foot and cross your right calf over your left.

② Roll up and down from your calf to your ankle. Do 20 strokes up and down.

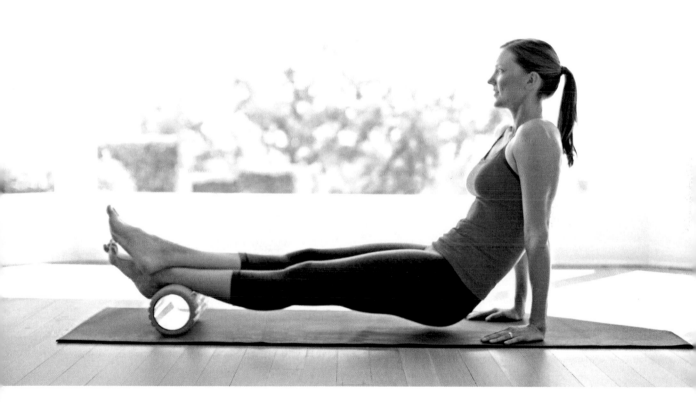

3 Rotate your leg out and roll on the outside of your calf. Do 20 strokes in that position.

4 Turn your leg in and roll on the inside of your calf. Do 20 strokes in that position.

Repeat on the other side.

HAMSTRINGS

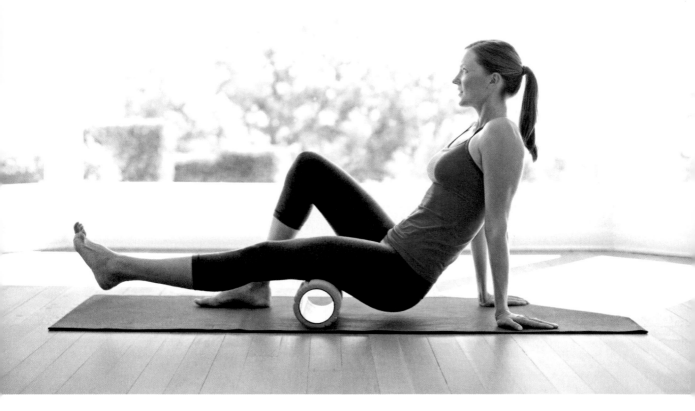

1 Sit with the roller under your left thigh with your right leg bent. Lean back with straight arms, supporting your weight with your hands.

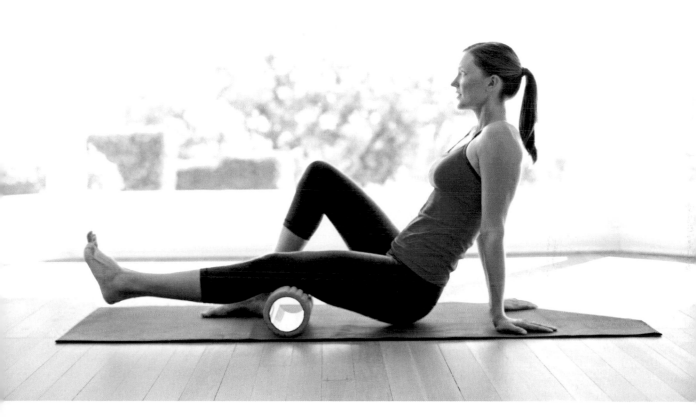

2 Roll up and down from the bottom of your hip to your knee 20 times.

3 Rotate your leg out and roll on the outside of your hamstring 20 times.

4 Turn your leg in and roll on the inside of your hamstring 20 times.

Repeat on the other side.

ADDUCTOR

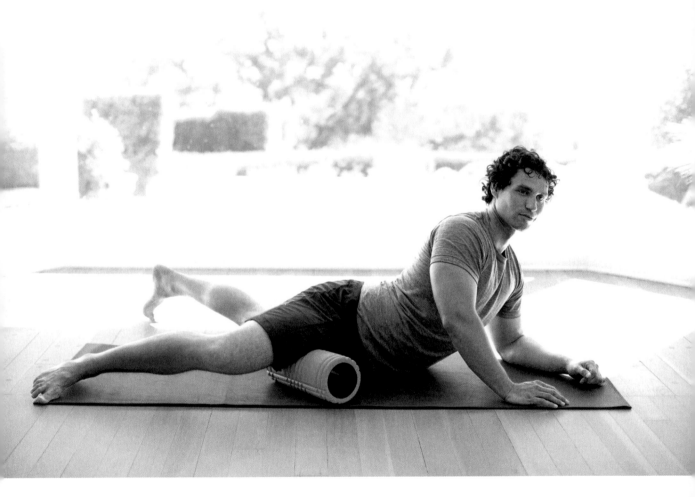

1 Lie facedown on the floor, then raise your upper body on your hands and forearms.

2 Extend your right leg over the roller.

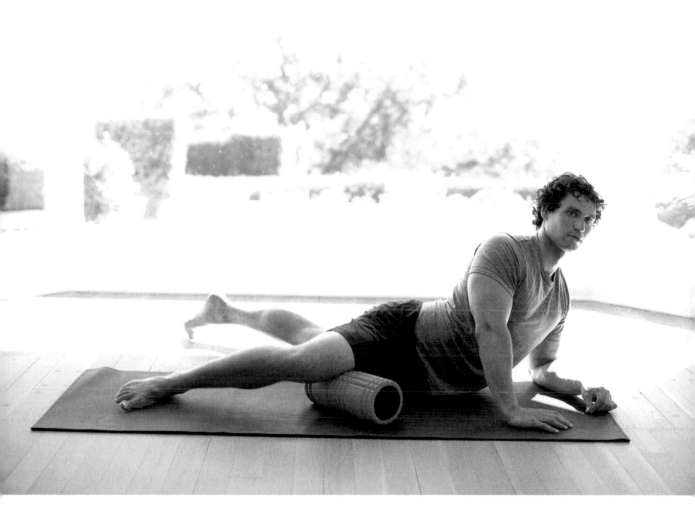

3 Roll on the inside of your thigh from the top of your thigh to your knee 20 times.

Repeat on the other side.

IT BAND

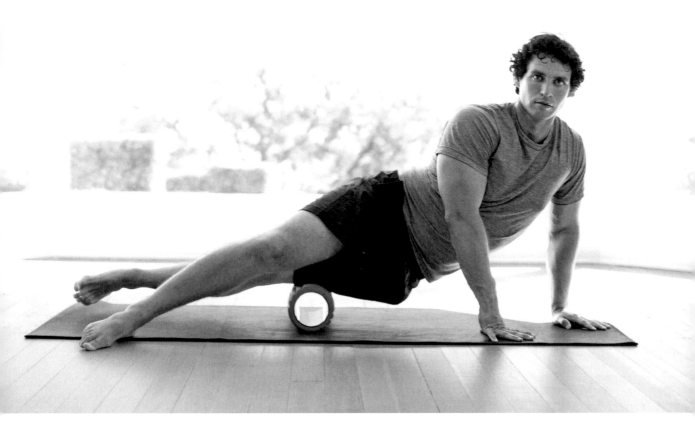

1 Lie on your right side with your bottom leg extended and the foam roller at your knee.

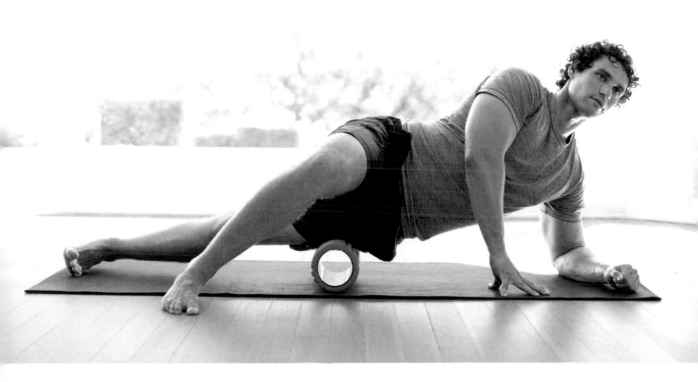

2 Cross your left leg over the bottom leg and put your left foot on the floor.

3 Roll up the side of your thigh to your hip bone and back down 20 times.

Repeat on the other side.

GLUTES

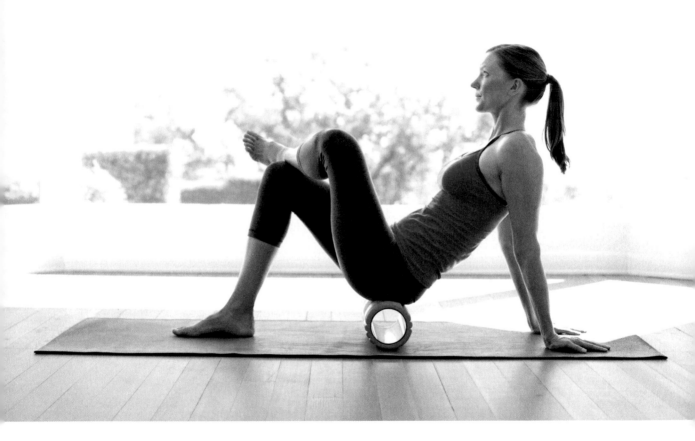

1 Sit on the foam roller with your left leg crossed over your right knee and your right foot flat on the ground. Put your hands on the floor behind you.

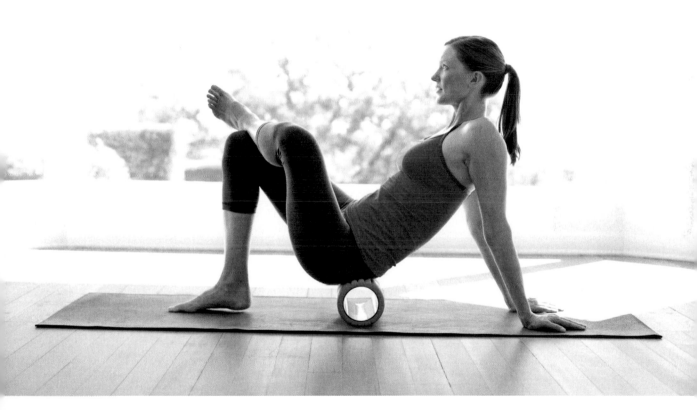

2 Roll from your butt to your lower hip 20 times.

Repeat on the other side.

QUADS

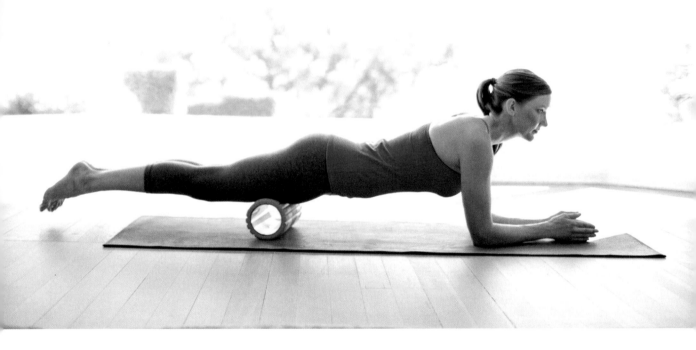

1 Lie facedown with the foam roller under your right thigh above your kneecap. Support your body weight with your hands or forearms.

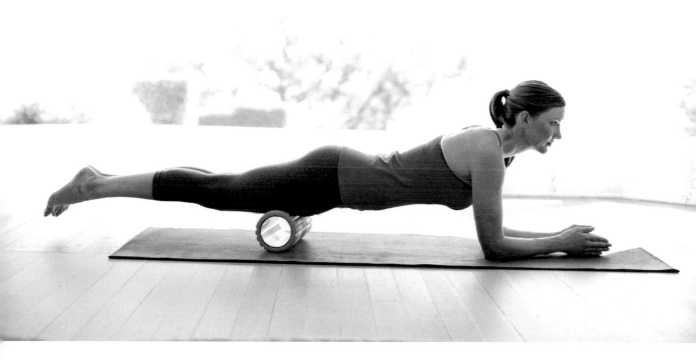

2 Roll up the front of your thigh to the bottom of your hip 20 times.

3 Roll on the outside of your quads 20 times.

4 Roll on the inside of your quads 20 times.

Repeat on the other side.

PSOAS—HIP FLEXORS

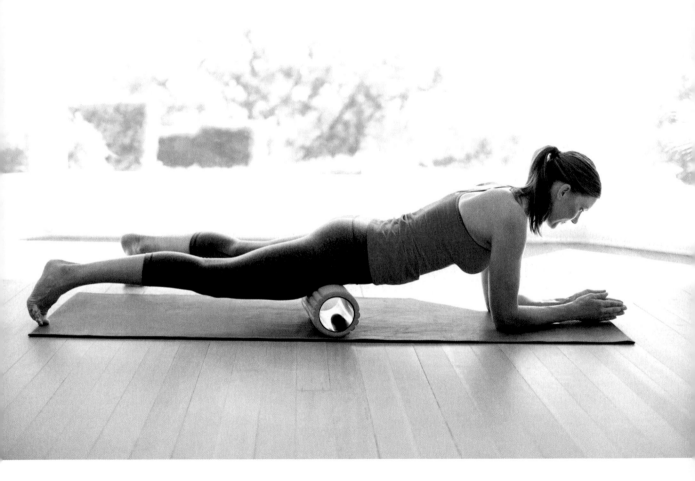

1 Lie facedown on the floor with the foam roller at the top of your right thigh. Support your body weight with your hands and forearms.

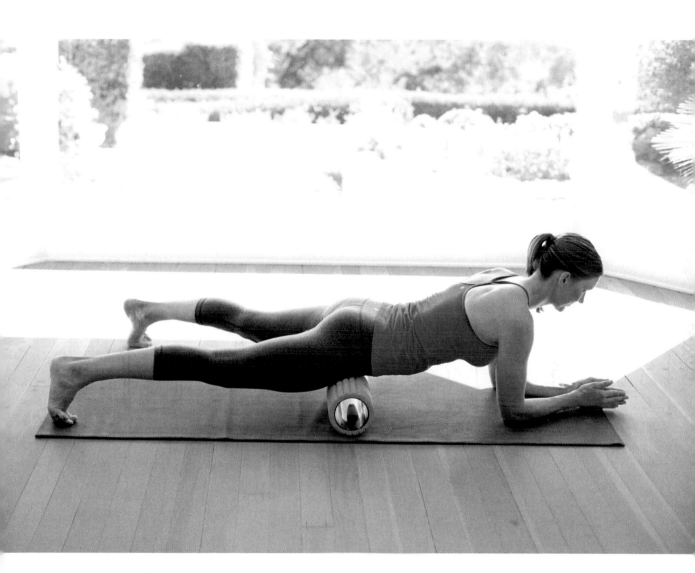

2 Roll up to the top of your hip bone and down 20 times.

Repeat on the other side.

LATS

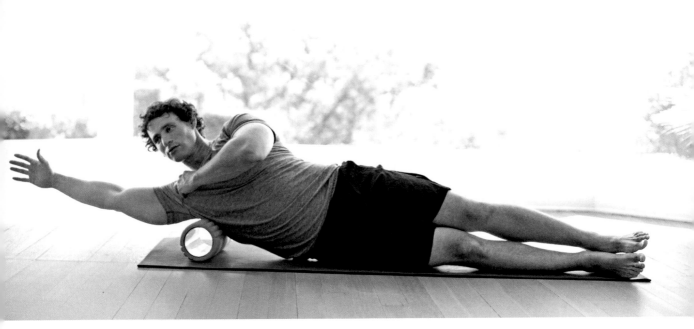

1 Lie on your right side and extend your bottom arm.

2 Put the roller horizontally below your chest.

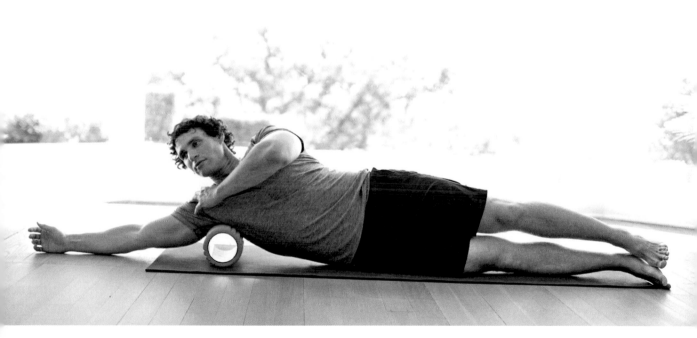

3 Roll up just past your armpit and shoulder and back down to your chest 20 times.

Repeat on the other side.

PECS

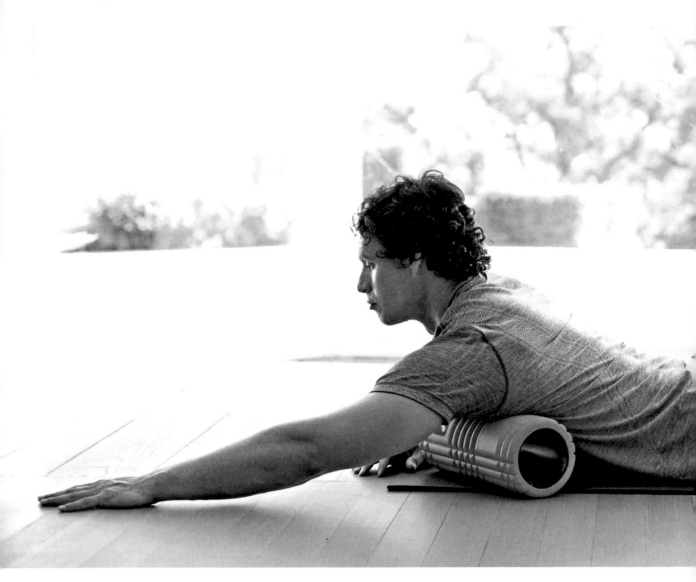

1 Lie on your stomach, your left arm extended and the foam roller under your armpit at the top of your chest.

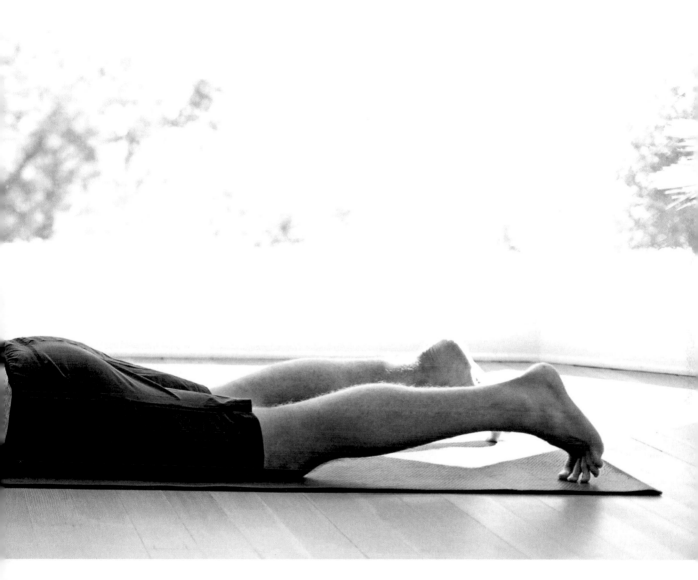

2 Roll up and down on your pecs 20 times.

Repeat on the other side.

UPPER SPINE

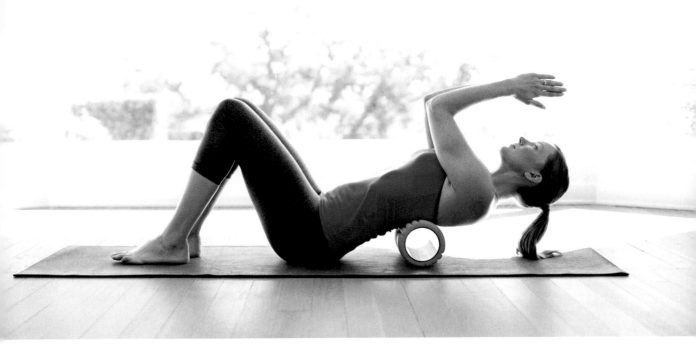

1 Put the foam roller at your midback and lie down on it, placing your feet arm's length from your butt. Press your palms together a few inches in front of your face.

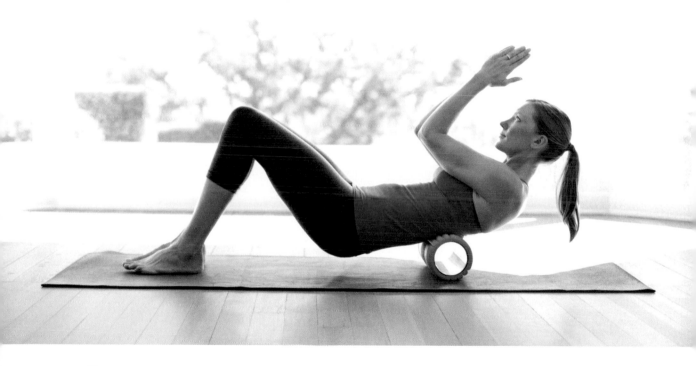

2 Lift your hips off the floor and roll toward the top of your back and down to the middle 20 times.

LOWER SPINE

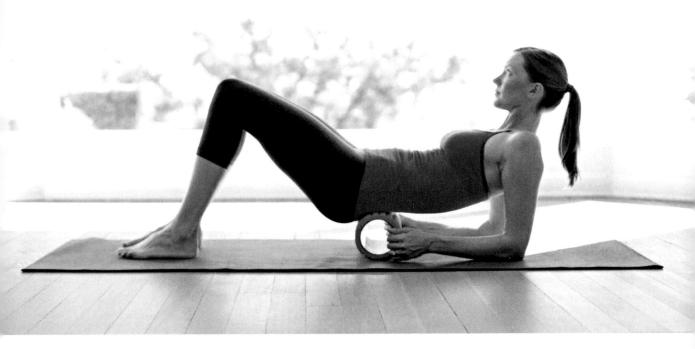

1 Lie on your back with the foam roller just above your glutes.

2 Raise yourself on bent elbows.

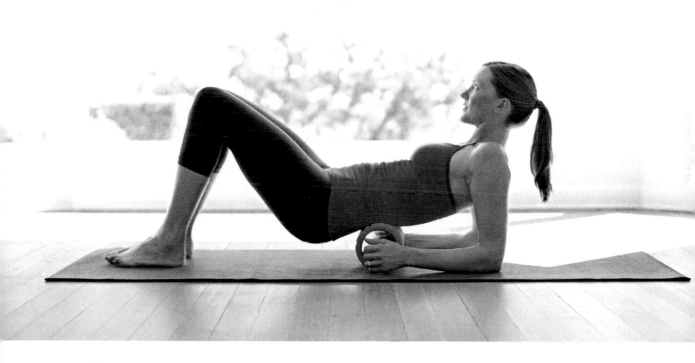

3 Roll up to your waist and down 20 times.

You might prefer to use a tennis ball for an active release of knots in smaller areas. Use the ball in the same way you would use the foam roller, using your body weight for an active release. Just put the ball of your choice where your muscle is tightest and roll away. This works particularly well with the glutes and the calves.

ARCHES

Don't forget your feet, which take a lot of beating supporting your weight.

1 Place the arch of your foot on a ball and roll it back and forth 20 times.

Repeat on the other foot.

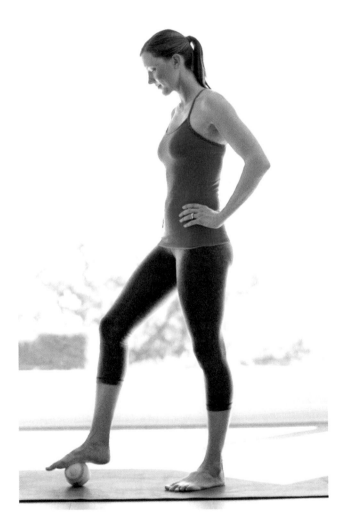

TOES

Women who wear high heels often have problems with cramps in their toes. And a long, hard run can compress your toes regardless of how comfortable your running shoes are. These foot massages feel great after a long run or after spending a lot of time on your feet.

1 Curl your toes around a ball and hold for 20 seconds.

2 Flex your toes, put them on the ball, and press down for 20 seconds.

Repeat five times.

Do the same on the other foot.

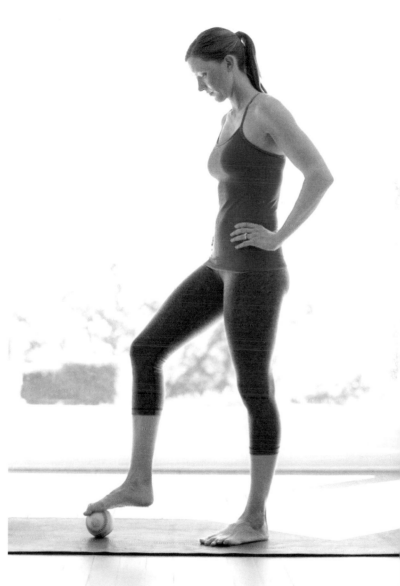

AFTERWORD

ONWARD AND UPWARD

We've said it before, and we'll say it again—you can take Foundation training as far as you want and apply the new movement patterns you have learned to any physical activity you decide to pursue. The first 6 weeks of Foundation training is the initial builder. It is a training program you can intensify as you get stronger. Now that you have restored your ability to move with freedom and power, the idea of falling back to old, inactive habits or not challenging yourself physically should be unthinkable. You have learned and felt what proper movement can do for you.

When you are feeling great, you want to keep feeling that way. You will do what you have to do to stay as fit as you can. That does not mean becoming a fanatic and going over the top. You know that a big component of the Foundation lifestyle is rest and restoration. Foundation training brings your body back into balance, and that should carry over mentally as well. When you are pain free, the work opens up to you again, and your priorities become clear. Doing things that are good for you becomes a way of life.

We are realistic about back pain and cannot promise that you will never feel a twinge or an ache in your back again. Stress, overexertion, a long airplane flight, sleeping the wrong way—any number of things can aggravate existing back prob-lems. But you do have the tools to handle any pain that comes you way. We begin our own workouts with the Founder at the very least to activate the posterior chain and reinforce keeping our backs extended.

We would be very interested to hear about your experience with Foundation training: how easy you found the exercises to learn, how you felt while you were learning them, what improvements you saw, how soon you felt a change. Please let us know how Foundation training worked for you. You can contact us through our Web site, www.foundationroots.com.

You can refer to the Web site as a supplement to the book. You can see what Foundation training is doing for others and hear the latest from us.

We know your experience with Foundation training will inspire the people around you. We hope you, as our clients have done, will pass it on, letting people know that this simple workout can change their lives.

Be good to your body, and it will serve you well.

ACKNOWLEDGMENTS

Thank you to my family, friends, clients, and teachers who have helped keep me on an interesting path in life and for humoring me when I talked a bit too much about the way we are supposed to move.

As a chiropractor, Tom Hyde, DC, has improved the education of countless healers and the lives of so many patients. As a friend, Tom has introduced me to opportunities to advance my education and experience as a person. For current and future practitioners, Tom has helped create the treatment protocol FAKTR-PM, which is advancing the way people treat musculoskeletal injuries.

Terry Schroeder, DC, and the US men's water polo team: The time I spent with you changed what I believed was possible and gave me the confidence to follow this dream. The dedication and effort these athletes put into preparing for an Olympic year is unbelievable. Thank you for the opportunity of a lifetime.

Diane Reverand, thank you for your guidance and patience throughout the entire process. Without your help we would still be on page 4.

David Vigliano, thank you for believing in *Foundation* and creating this opportunity.

Senior editor Shannon Welch, Stephanie Knapp, Chris Rhoads, Karen Rinaldi, Colin Dickerman, Emily Weber, and Zachary Greenwald for not only making this book but for making us feel like part of the Rodale family every time we were in New York.

Scott Holladay, your illustrations brought this book to the next level.

Peter Park, your inexhaustible desire to learn is the reason this book happened as soon as it did and with as much momentum as it did. You inspire so many people by living what you teach. Thank you for embracing *Foundation*, putting your reputation and energy behind it and introducing your world to this work.

Thank you again to my friends and family for everlasting love and support.

—ERIC GOODMAN

To my incredible and supportive family and my loving wife, Kelly, who always points me in the right direction and is always by my side supporting me in whatever I do. To my two kids, Hayden and Carter, who mean everything to me and keep me happier than I ever thought possible.

To Lance Armstrong, whose friendship and association have opened doors to further my career to levels I never imagined. Your hard work, energy, and dedication to everything you do inspire me.

To Casey Wasserman, a true friend who has been there whenever I needed him. Without him, this book would not have been possible.

To Barry Cappello, my first client and a huge influence in my life for over 20 years.

To Tim Brown, DC, a great mentor whose principles and ideas have influenced me greatly.

To Eric Goodman, whose knowledge and ideas have made me approach training in an entirely different way. In Eric, I have found an individual who shares my passion for the truth. I am lucky and honored to have formed this partnership. We have gone so far so fast; I cannot wait to see what we can accomplish in the future!

—PETER PARK

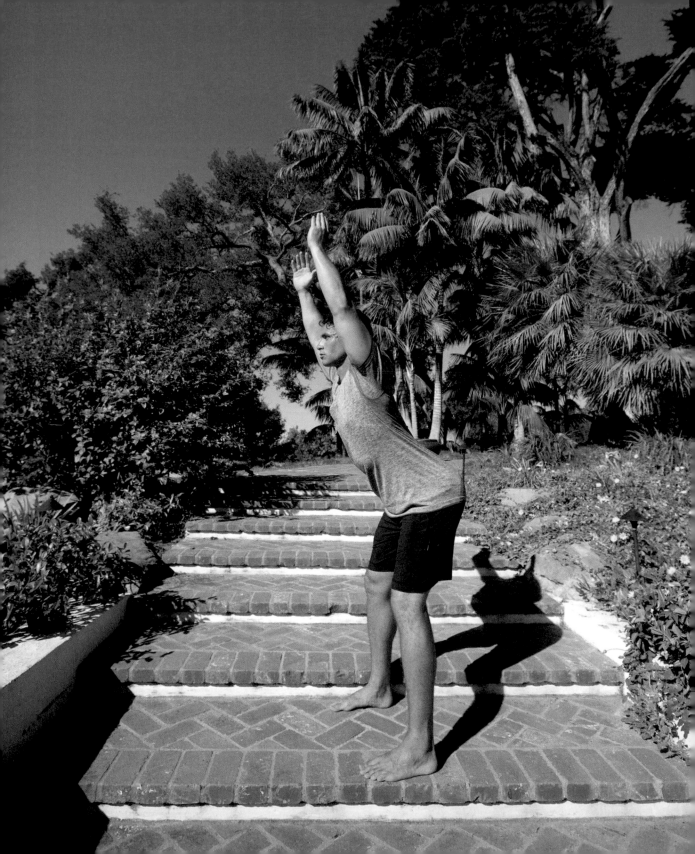

ONLINE RESOURCES

Find more information about Foundation training, including videos and testimonials.

www.foundationroots.com

Peter's gym, Platinum Fitness, provides goal-oriented, performance-driven plans to suit everyone's needs.

www.sbplatinumfitness.com

Lance Armstrong Foundation built LIVESTRONG.com as the definitive daily health, fitness, and lifestyle destination.

www.livestrong.com

Tim Brown, DC, developed Intelliskin—postural apparel that is second to none and complements Foundation training better than anything else available.

www.intelliskinusa.com

FAKTR-PM stands for Functional and Kinetic Treatment with Rehabilitation, Provocation, and Motion. It was developed to help speed recovery from chronic musculoskeletal pain syndromes and has also been shown to work extremely well on acute musculoskeletal/fascial conditions.

www.faktr-pm.com

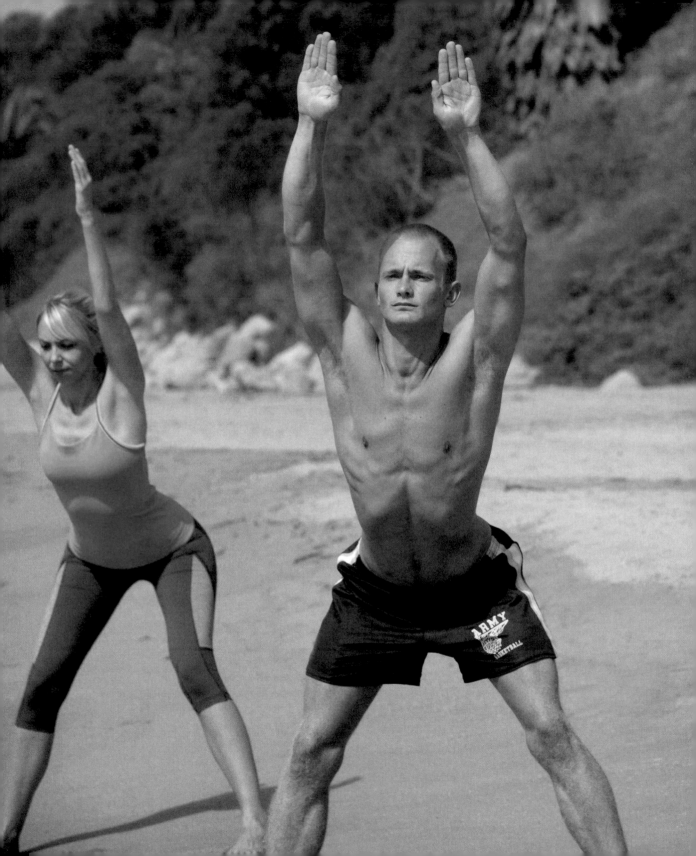

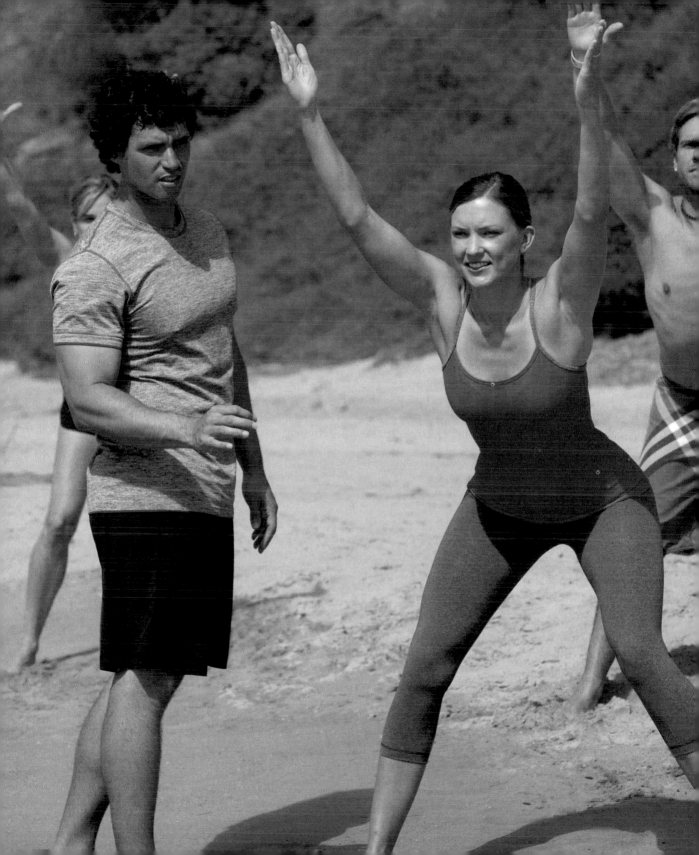

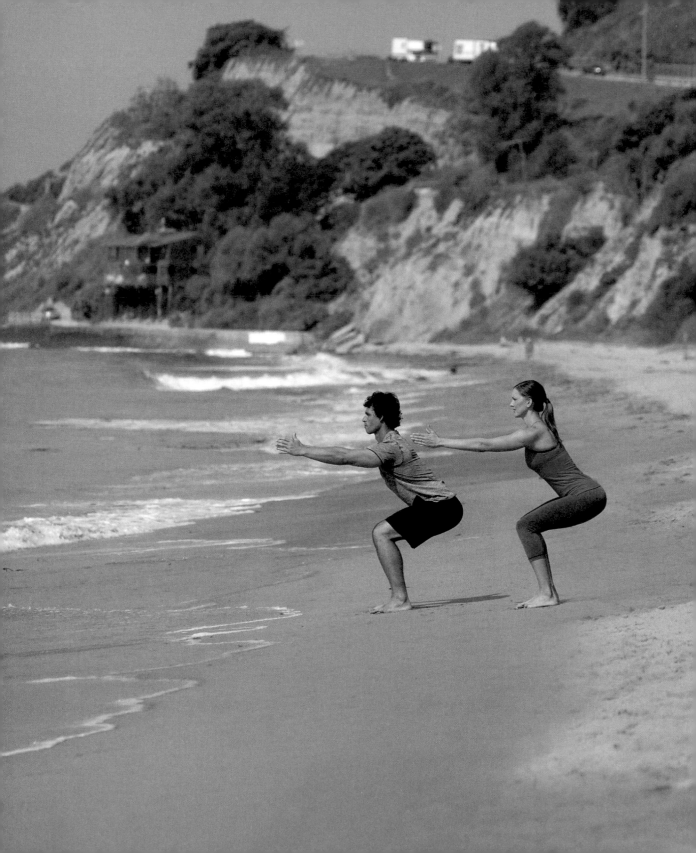

INDEX

Boldface page references indicate illustrations. <u>Underscored</u> references indicate boxed text.